The
GOOD
DEATH

The
GOOD
DEATH

A GUIDE for SUPPORTING YOUR LOVED ONE THROUGH the END of LIFE

SUZANNE B. O'BRIEN, RN

LITTLE, BROWN SPARK
New York Boston London

This book is dedicated to all the family caregivers who will be called to care for someone they love at the end of life.

May this book bring you empowerment, comfort, and guidance for the most peaceful passing possible.

Contents

The
GOOD
DEATH

Introduction

Don't be afraid of death; be afraid of an
unlived life. You don't have to live forever,
you just have to live.

—Natalie Babbitt in *Tuck Everlasting*

grabbed the cold, stainless steel handle of the door to hospital
room 575 and entered. It looked exactly like every other hospital
room I had been in over the course of my nursing career. The
same reflective linoleum flooring, the same perforated ceiling tiles,
and the same off-white walls. It was sterile in every way—just as
void of vibrancy and warmth as it was void of bacteria.

But when I entered room 575 that particular day, I felt something different. There were four family members gathered around
the bedside, looking at my patient. She was unconscious, her
breathing shallow and labored. I stood behind them, silently
observing. The only sounds were the slow beeps coming from the
electronic vital signs monitor and the rhythmic whooshing of the
IV pump.

The patient's mouth was slightly agape. I immediately knew I
was witnessing the end of this woman's life. She was actively transitioning into death.

I was accustomed to witnessing a state of crisis, panic, and fear
in moments like these. After all, death is the number one fear in the

United States (and probably almost everywhere else on the planet). But in this moment, I felt no fear in the room. There was only calm.

Then, I felt something powerful around me. It was as if I was watching her spirit leave the physical world behind and ascend elsewhere. I was accustomed to witnessing death, but I had never seen anything like this. An incommunicable feeling of love enveloped the room, and for a moment, it felt like time had disappeared. I stood there in complete awe.

The experience was peaceful all the way through to her final breath, and when she transitioned, I quietly left the room so that her loved ones could say their goodbyes in private. As I closed that stainless steel door behind me, my eyes filled with tears of gratitude for what I had just been allowed to witness.

At that point, I had worked in end-of-life care as a registered nurse for one and a half years. After eighteen months of witnessing death on a daily basis, this was the first time I ever saw what I would characterize as a "good death." All the other times, I watched my patients and their families suffer physically and emotionally until death inevitably came, throwing everyone into traumatic grief.

That day, I realized that as a society, the relationship we have with death is all wrong. Death doesn't have to be scary, and our fear of it is misguided. I understood then that it can be a beautiful and profound experience for all involved, and I knew if people could see what I had just seen, they wouldn't be so afraid anymore.

That day was so different from what I usually experienced that it left an indelible mark on my consciousness. I had come from a medical family. My father was a doctor, and my mother worked in hospital administration. My whole life, I heard about patients dying and the importance of showing them compassion. Then, when I dreamed of my own career as a nurse, I pictured myself helping my patients manage both their pain and their fears, helping them get through some of the most difficult experiences of their lives. I envisioned a rewarding career that allowed me to give back and provide real comfort to others. Unfortunately, my first job on the medical surgical floor of a hospital was a far cry from that vision.

The reality was that I wasn't given enough time with my patients to truly provide the care they needed. Despite working fourteen-hour shifts, my average time with a patient wasn't long enough to be present with them. I was too busy getting the initial report, assessing their situation, giving medications, making notes on their chart, and then moving to the next person. I felt like a robotic medical machine. The compassionate care I longed to give my patients seemed out of reach.

I couldn't help but notice the high number of elderly patients who were regularly admitted. They would come in through the emergency medical service, often connected to tubes and machines. It wasn't uncommon for them to spend days or even weeks in their hospital rooms. What struck me most was that many of them had no visitors. They were barely awake, and some died alone in those sterile rooms.

I yearned for more time to spend with all of my patients, but especially the elderly ones. I wanted to hold their hands, speak softly to them, and let them know they weren't alone. But in the fast-paced world of medical care, that kind of time simply didn't exist.

As my frustrations grew in my career, I felt a deep longing to go into hospice nursing. Despite not having any end-of-life care experience at that point, I believed that supporting patients and their families during this precious time was my true calling. I knew that society shied away from open conversations about death, but surely in hospice care, where end-of-life support was provided, I could offer *holistic* care. I believed I could discuss death openly and create an environment for a peaceful end of life. But again, once I began working in hospice care, I saw that the reality was something else entirely. While people expected their loved one in hospice care to die, thus somewhat reducing the panic and fear, medical practitioners were still not given enough time with them to facilitate a good death.

Over an eleven-year period, I worked with elderly patients in a hospital setting, followed by work as a hospice nurse and an oncology nurse. I can confidently say that during my time in hospice— just like my time in hospitals—nine out of ten times, my patients' deaths didn't go as well as they could have.

The truth is that most end-of-life care is provided by family members, but they aren't given instructions on what to do or how to handle the challenges they will face. Most home hospice nurses are given an average of sixty minutes per week to teach the family how to care for someone who is on their way to dying. It isn't nearly enough, so my frustrations only intensified.

THE BIRTH OF DOULAGIVERS

As I became more and more disheartened by barriers to the care I was able to provide as a hospice worker, I sat down and developed a three-phase process to teach families how to care for their loved ones at the end of life (which has been incorporated within this book in chapter 3). I decided to take my three-phase process to the administrator of the facility where I was working at the time. "We're supposed to teach families how to care for their loved ones, but it isn't going well," I told him. "I have an idea for a training." I proceeded to explain to him what I had created.

"This is great!" he said. "But you can't do it."

My heart sank. "Why not?" I asked.

"Because insurance won't reimburse for it."

Ouch. Bureaucracy was in the way.

Nevertheless, I refused to let that stop me. I decided to offer my training at a local library for free on a Saturday and see what would happen. The very first training, there wasn't an empty seat in the room. At least fifty people attended, including a man who told the group that his son had just been diagnosed with pancreatic cancer. "I want to learn everything I can to help him," he said.

At the end of the training, that man was beaming. He felt empowered because he had some understanding of how to be there for his son during the hardest time either of them would ever experience. He had a plan, and clearly that gave him immense comfort in the face of terrible grief.

That day, I realized people were hungry for this information, but I wouldn't know to what extent that was true until I put the training online. Suddenly, people all over the world were clamoring for it. When I began giving webinars online, I learned that there were people on the other side of the world who were staying up until 2:00 a.m. or 5:00 a.m. to make sure they didn't miss it.

I had found a way to empower more people to help their loved ones have a good death. Before long, I founded the International Doulagivers Institute and became its CEO. We offer the highest level of education and certification for full-spectrum, holistic, non-medical end-of-life care practitioners known as "Doulagivers." Our state-of-the-art Professional Certification Program teaches "death doulas" to guide patients and families through the entire end-of-life journey, providing support before, during, and after death. Besides our Professional Certification Program, we also offer a free Level 1 End-of-Life Doula and Family Caregiver Training, helping family members know how to care for their loved ones at end of life. Each month, between 2,500 and 5,000 people register and attend this online webinar training from all around the world. As of this writing, the organization has trained more than 360,000 people across thirty-four countries.

And this book you're reading right now is the next step in getting the word out about how to facilitate a good death for the people you cherish so much. It's a step-by-step, definitive guide to helping your loved one have a good death not just physically, but also emotionally, mentally, spiritually, and financially.

WHAT YOU WILL LEARN

If you have picked up this book, I assume either you are already in the throes of dealing with the impending loss of someone dear to you, or you are perhaps thinking ahead, wanting to be prepared for when that day might come. Either way, you want to ease the suffering of your loved one as much as you possibly can, while also easing your own suffering and the pain your family and friends might feel. I'm here to tell you that the beautiful experience I described at the beginning of the book is possible for you, but you need information to facilitate it. This book is designed to give you that comprehensive information and help you understand exactly what it means to have a *good death*.

While these chapters have been written primarily for the caregiver of someone who is at the end of life, they can also be used by anyone who wants to prepare for their own death. I also want to note that my experience has been in the United States, and there will be some differences as to specifics if you live in a different country. But through Doulagivers, I have worked with people all over the globe and found that there are many commonalities we all share when faced with the end of life.

Here is what you will learn as you continue reading:

Part 1: Facilitating a Good Death

Chapter 1: We Become Less Fearful of the Unknown When We Embrace What Is Known. We tend to be fearful of what we don't understand. While no one knows for sure what happens after we die, this chapter is aimed toward helping you understand death a bit better, such as the natural ways in which the body systematically shuts down no matter who we are, where we live, or what our socioeconomic status/belief system is.

Chapter 2: Preparing for Longer Lifespans: The Elder Care Crisis. Life expectancy has nearly doubled over the last century, and we have to prepare for that. This chapter will teach you what you need to know about Living Well Aging Plans, advance directives, and more.

Chapter 3: How to Care for Someone Who Is Dying: The Three Phases of End of Life. Throughout my years of service in this field, I have identified three distinct phases of end of life and the interventions that assist us in getting through each of them. I will cover what can be done to help the dying person, the caregiver, and other loved ones so they may move through each phase with as much comfort and ease as possible.

Chapter 4: Dealing with Common Diseases at End of Life. Knowing what to expect when your loved one has a particular disease will help you care for them better and feel more confident every day. This chapter will provide guidelines for the most common life-threatening diseases that people face.

Chapter 5: How Caregivers Can Avoid Burnout. I have watched so many loving people care for others to the point of exhaustion. People would love to help you, but unless you know how to ask for it, they often don't know how to offer it. This chapter will help you avoid the traps of burnout.

Chapter 6: The Rebirth of Death. People today are going back to their roots with the readoption of home wakes and funerals. Centuries ago, this was the common way to handle death. In this chapter, I'll provide you with the various options available besides a "standard" funeral, as well as an exercise to explore plans for a memorial for your loved one and/or for yourself in the future.

Chapter 7: Keeping Death Green: How Our Funeral and Burial Choices Impact the Planet. We can still have a significant impact on the world even after death by making an informed and conscious decision to protect the environment with our burial choice. This chapter will include the growing movement toward rituals that embrace natural body disposition and natural burials.

Part 2: The Peace of Mind Planner

Chapters 8–12 make up the Peace of Mind Planner, which is a complete, practical, and holistic planning guide for end-of-life wishes for individuals and families. It includes the categories I have outlined as the most important during my time in hospice and in training other death doulas: physical, mental, emotional, financial, and spiritual. These chapters will address the concerns that people have expressed to me over my more than twenty years in this field. The planner includes worksheets that will set you and your loved one up for a good death in each of these areas, incorporating what you learned in chapters 1–7.

Chapter 8: A Physical Good Death. This chapter will provide all the choices and questions you need to address to help your loved one achieve a physical good death. What are their physical preferences and needs?

Chapter 9: A Mental Good Death. This chapter will cover how to find mental peace of mind at the end of life, including finding acceptance and calm when someone we love receives a terminal diagnosis.

Chapter 10: An Emotional Good Death. Here, you will learn the most common emotional pain points that you can expect to feel when facing end of life or losing a loved one. I will share the tools to create emotional peace around these pain points.

Chapter 11: A Financial Good Death. Since most families don't plan in advance, they end up spending far more money than necessary. When we do plan ahead, we can save our family and loved ones thousands, if not tens of thousands, of dollars. You will learn the options available so that you can plan for supporting your loved one in the most cost-effective way.

Chapter 12: A Spiritual Good Death. There's a moment during the end-of-life journey when a person has one foot in this world and one foot in the next. It's a sacred and healing moment that I describe as getting their "spiritual eyes." This chapter will prepare you for when this moment happens and what you can do to facilitate it.

Epilogue: Death as a Sacred Experience

In many cultures throughout history, death was honored and revered as an important phase of life. Today, unfortunately, we have lost this sacred connection to death, which can be our greatest teacher about life. In this final chapter, I will discuss ways that you can open yourself to experiencing the death of your loved one as a sacred experience, as well as ways to facilitate that experience for them.

I WILL HOLD YOUR HAND ON THIS JOURNEY

I know that you're facing something that is frightening and enormously painful. My aim with this book is to give you the comfort of having a plan and the knowledge to make this process of transitioning from life to death a beautiful, sacred, and profound experience for everyone involved. After my initial unfortunate experiences as a nurse, I have seen this kind of good death happen many, many times, and have taught countless others to facilitate such a death for others. I have seen the peace that it offers, not only to the person who is transitioning, but to the people who are left behind.

As you walk this path, allow me to hold your hand, figuratively speaking, through the words you will read on these pages.

PART 1

FACILITATING A GOOD DEATH

MANY OF US WILL HAVE to show up for someone we love at the end of life. Knowing how to do that changes everything. After working with more than one thousand people at end of life, I can confidently say that in my experience, planning ahead makes end of life dramatically better, no matter the disease process.

So in part 1, my goal is to give you the knowledge you need to make your loved one's transition as smooth as possible—not just for them, but for you and everyone involved. We'll start by addressing our fear of death head-on and look at how that fear has only made the end-of-life process harder.

We'll also talk about the kinds of documents your loved one will need to make sure their wishes are known ahead of time.

I'll take away the guesswork of caring for someone who is dying so that you know what to do and what to ask hospice nurses, including a rundown of the most common diseases you're likely to encounter.

I'll address *you* and what you need to do to make sure you don't overextend yourself and become exhausted by the caregiving experience. I'll also provide options for funerals, memorial services, and burials.

Caring for a loved one at this pivotal time may be the most moving and profound experience of your life. Let's make it easier!

1

We Become Less Fearful of the Unknown When We Embrace What Is Known

The most beautiful and profound emotion we
can experience is the sensation of the mystical.

—Albert Einstein

My patient, Vivian, was scheduled for exploratory surgery as her entire family gathered in her oncology ward hospital room, feeling a mixture of anxiety and hope. But when I examined her, I could see the tumors visibly protruding through the skin of her abdomen. There was no question that her intestinal cancer had reached an advanced stage.

Despite my efforts to find a suitable spot on her stomach to listen for bowel sounds with my stethoscope, I already knew the likelihood of detecting any was slim. The cancer had seized control of this elderly woman's body, and it was clear her life was nearing its end.

Yet, because of the fear of death and the lack of a truthful conversation between the family and the doctor, everyone involved pretended that death was either not happening or at least optional. As a result, Vivian's care went into "default" or what I call the "medical treadmill," subjecting her to a futile major surgical procedure that would only confirm what we already knew. I had no doubt the surgeon would see that the cancer was widespread in her body, and he would just close her back up because there was nothing more he could do. And that's exactly what happened.

For Vivian and her family, this was *not* a good death. It was a heart-wrenching, harrowing one. And time and again, this is what I saw in my career as a nurse.

Why were we offering false hope to this woman and her family? Why were we subjecting her to the rigors, pain, and recovery of an invasive surgery that would do her no good? Why does the medical field do this repeatedly?

Fueled by our society's intense fear of dying, our end-of-life care doesn't work well because we lack an understanding of the difference between keeping people alive and allowing them to live with quality of life. Instead, we expect doctors to somehow fix the unfixable and to defy the inevitable. In cases like Vivian's, there would always come a point when their efforts did more harm than good.

Clearly, our end-of-life care is dysfunctional, and this dysfunction is preventing most people from having a good death.

In this chapter, let's talk about this fear, how it makes end of life even harder, and how we can begin to quell it by learning more about what happens as we near death. In other words, we can become less fearful of death if we embrace what we *do* know about it.

WHY ARE WE SO AFRAID?

Has the language we use within the medical system inadvertently contributed to our subconscious war with death? We speak of "losing battles" against illnesses, urging patients to fight. And when all options have been exhausted, we apologize for our inability to offer further assistance. In this relentless fight, it seems that death has become the ultimate adversary. Regardless of our wishes or efforts, it's an enemy that will always emerge victorious in the end, despite countless treatments, procedures, and surgeries. We cannot beat it. And even though we can sometimes postpone it, does it truly make sense to do that at all costs regardless of the quality of life during the time we have left? While doctors should certainly do what they can, there does come that moment when letting go and accepting the inevitable would be the most compassionate choice for the patient, the patient's loved ones, and also for the doctor.

As an oncology nurse, I have witnessed overwhelming fear of death in my patients, in their loved ones, and in medical professionals. It has become clear to me that this fear often leads to misguided decisions and unnecessary procedures and treatments that cause more pain, discomfort, and side effects in patients who still ultimately succumb to their illnesses.

Perhaps the real source of our fear is the fact that we have stripped death of its natural place in the journey of life. By trying to shield ourselves from it and by using language that reinforces our fears, we may have unknowingly nurtured an unjustified dread about this sacred and integral part of life's progression.

Our unhealthy fear prevents us from having necessary conversations about the end of life and from embracing the timeless wisdom death can offer us. This fear prevents us from caring for each other in a way that lessens the suffering and increases the quality of life of all involved, while maintaining the dignity of the patient.

It hasn't always been like this. In the distant past, the way we cared for those who were dying wasn't as dysfunctional as it is now. It's important that we look back for a vision of how we might move forward with more grace and less fear.

HOW DID WE GET HERE?

Up until about a hundred years ago, caring for the dying was a skill passed down through generations from grandparents to their children and grandchildren. Death was embraced by rituals that allowed loved ones and communities to gather together and comfort each other toward the end.

When illness struck, people were historically cared for in the comfort of their own homes. They died surrounded by loved ones, and their wakes were even held in the home. People who came to the house to pay their respects congregated in the "living room" before entering the parlor, where the deceased was laid out for viewing. This is why we all have a "living room" in our homes.

With the progression of science, however, death has become increasingly medicalized, stripping away its humanity. With the advancements of modern medicine, life expectancy in the US soared from about forty-eight years in 1900 to about eighty years today.[1] Worldwide, life expectancy was only thirty-two years in 1900 and increased to seventy-one years by 2021.[2] While this is undoubtedly a remarkable achievement that we all benefit from, it has also brought about significant changes in the way we approach death.

Families are left feeling disempowered as medical systems take control and send the terminally ill to medical institutions designed to treat and cure ailments even when it's clear the end is near. Modern medicine's primary focus is to keep people breathing at all costs, but those costs are great—and not just financial. One of those costs is that concentrating on keeping people alive means we fail to provide the support that those transitioning out of this world truly need.

Since medical school is designed to equip doctors with the skills to prolong life, there are generally no courses on the topic of death. During their education, medical students endure demanding schedules, rigorous classes, and extensive internships with long hours. This grueling process, lasting anywhere from six to ten years depending on their chosen specialty, leaves little room for "outside the box" thinking. It's no wonder that doctors are set up for inevitable failure when it comes to appropriately treating death and the dying. It's an unfair burden for them to bear. After all, they are human, too.

The current fragmented health care system fails to allocate enough time for discussions about end-of-life care, and doctors are not trained for those discussions. Instead, they are constrained by strict time limits when interacting with patients, sometimes as little as fifteen minutes. Informing someone and their family of a terminal diagnosis, along with the impossibility of reversing the disease, can't be condensed into such a short conversation. And when it is, it's unbearably insensitive.

Of course, this is a symptom of our societal lack of awareness about death and lack of willingness to discuss it openly, as well as the fact that doctors are often perceived as failures if their patients die, *regardless of age or diagnosis*. All of this leads doctors to avoid broaching the subject altogether. It would be much more compassionate for all involved if health care providers felt they could be transparent about the limitations of aggressive treatments when the chances of disease reversal are minimal at best. People like Vivian would then be spared painful surgeries that medical professionals know are pointless but feel obligated to perform; this medical treadmill has become the norm since there is no conversation about death between the patient, family, and doctor.

In end-of-life health care, there is a delicate balance between being helpful and potentially causing harm. The question is: *Who should decide where that line is drawn?*

In my opinion, responsibility for end-of-life care lies with both the individual and their health care providers. It's crucial for people to reflect on their own values and preferences, determining what quality of life means for them personally. To ensure these wishes are honored, it's essential to document them in advance directives (which we will discuss in the next chapter) and talk about them openly with family members and doctors.

To do this, we must get past our aversion to accepting the inevitable. When we talk about death frankly and compassionately without pretending that doctors can work miracles, we save ourselves a lot of pain in the future.

For example, Alice was a ninety-three-year-old woman with advanced breast cancer in my hospital's oncology unit. Despite her frailty and failing health, she didn't have a do not resuscitate (DNR) order in place.

As a nurse familiar with end-of-life situations, I could foresee that she was close to a critical point. Her lab numbers were declining, she appeared pale and unresponsive, and her journey with cancer was nearing its end. But without a DNR order, I was legally obligated to perform cardiopulmonary resuscitation (CPR) if her heart stopped. CPR was originally developed to save healthy individuals who experienced sudden cardiac arrest. It has since become a standard procedure in all health care situations, including terminal ones like Alice's. This raises the question of its purpose and the quality of life that sometimes results.

Performing CPR on Alice would have involved breaking her ribs and potentially placing her on a machine to keep her alive—a machine that she would undoubtedly be unable to survive without. This would leave her family with the eventual decision of whether or when to turn off the machine. What kind of life would that be when death was still inevitable in a short period of time?

In my role in the oncology unit, I would often inform the doctors when I believed a patient was nearing the end, and I would advocate for an honest discussion with the family about signing a DNR order if one was not already in place. Of course, I knew these conversations would have been so much kinder and less stressful if held way before someone was admitted to the hospital.

In Alice's case, the doctor eventually recognized the need for a DNR order and was able to obtain the family's signature. The following day, she died peacefully with her loved ones by her side and with her dignity and ribs still intact. It was a good death. What if that could be our ultimate goal rather than striving for a breathing body? If the problem lies in the unrealistic expectation of prolonging life at all costs, perhaps managing expectations is the solution.

Could withholding honesty about someone's impending death be part of the harm that doctors have taken an oath not to do? I know of one instance when a woman's mother had gone through numerous cancer surgeries. An oncologist told her, "From a scientist's point of view, I could tell you to try this next surgery for your mother. But as a human being, I'm going to tell you to go home and make her comfortable."

In my opinion, it's time to bring back the awareness that *death is not a medical experience—it's a human one.*

THE HOSPICE GAP

If hospitals are problematic because of the insistence on keeping people alive no matter what and the lack of transparency around death, are hospice facilities the solution? After all, death is expected there, and comfort is considered key. People receive nonstop care there, right?

By definition, hospice care is considered to be the model for quality, compassionate care for people facing a serious or life-limiting illness or injury. It involves a team-oriented approach to expert medical care, pain management, and emotional and spiritual support for the patient and their loved ones, all expressly tailored to the patient's needs and wishes. In the US, health care providers use Medicare guidelines to determine eligibility for hospice care, and according to Medicare, someone is eligible if their life expectancy is six months or less if their illness were to run its natural course. Some of the most common diseases that qualify for hospice services are ALS, Alzheimer's disease/dementia, cancer, heart disease, kidney disease, and Parkinson's disease. It's a beautiful model...*in theory.*

Unfortunately, there are very few hospice facilities in the US that offer twenty-four-hour care. Because the majority of hospices today are for-profit businesses, and the Medicare hospice benefit pays a fixed per diem rate regardless of the quality of care provided, the ones that exist have few beds and are often understaffed.

The circumstances aren't much better in other parts of the world.

While the majority of countries have some form of hospice care, few have enough available beds for the growing numbers of elderly patients. Sadly, therefore, it isn't an option for many people.

Well, then, is the solution to send the dying home? Yes, since nine out of ten people say in polls that they would like to be at home if they become terminally ill. The problem, however, is that family members are expected to provide around-the-clock care without proper training. As someone with years of experience in home hospice care, I have all too often seen tragic situations created by a combination of fear and lack of caregiving knowledge. But the problem is that home hospice workers aren't given enough time to train family members properly. So there is a gap between the time required at the bedside of patients and what can be fulfilled by overtaxed hospice workers.

Where does that leave you? It leaves you with a book like this, which will give you all the tools you'll need for when you're faced with caring for someone who is nearing the end of their life. You will also learn a myriad of ways to be prepared so that you can ensure a good death for your loved one and be prepared for what you will face after their death.

Again, this includes making informed decisions about the kind of care they would want or not want in the final stages of life. When we think about it ahead of time and have a plan, fear doesn't hijack the experience from us and deny us the space to spend quality time with this person we love so much. Whether this window of time goes well or poorly, we'll remember it forever. A positive memory is what we want, and it's the kind of final experience we want for our loved ones. That's what a good death affords us. With that in mind, let's talk about some of the potential decisions that can ensure the dignity of the dying.

PALLIATIVE SEDATION

"Palliative" means that the treatment relieves symptoms but doesn't cure the illness. It's used to make people comfortable when their illness can't be cured.

Every year, millions of people are unable to resolve their physical, psychological, and spiritual suffering at the end of their lives. In fact, the World Health Organization (WHO) says that each year an estimated 25.7 million people at end of life need palliative care, but only about 14 percent of them actually receive it. Considering the amount of intolerable pain a person can face, palliative care is so important. Yet WHO cites unnecessarily restrictive regulations throughout the world for access to medicines that would reduce pain. It says, "The global need for palliative care will continue to grow as a result of the ageing of populations."[3]

Palliative sedation (also sometimes called terminal sedation, continuous deep sedation, palliative coma, or sedation for intractable distress of a dying patient) is a means of administering ongoing medication to keep the dying person asleep and comfortable. It's a last resort for people at end of life who are in a lot of pain, and it's administered to the terminally ill patient in the last days or hours of their life. It can provide a more peaceful and ethical solution for someone in this situation. (Note that there is also something called a "sleeping coma," which often happens naturally as a person nears the end of life. A "palliative coma," on the other hand, is a sleeping coma that has been facilitated by medication.)

If the person is in a hospital or hospice facility, it's usually administered intravenously. Other methods include (1) a sedative drug infused under the skin, (2) a specialized catheter via the rectum, (3) medication taken under the tongue, or (4) patches on the skin.

This type of sedation can be done at home. In fact, I have seen better control of pain in the home than in the hospital. This is because nurses have so many patients, and although they try hard, they will inevitably be spread thin. If medication needs to be increased to ease someone's pain, there's usually a hospital protocol that can delay it. In the home, on the other hand, family members are focused on one person and can monitor them more carefully.

The harsh reality is that the progression of pain must be broken on its way up when it reaches a level of 3 or 4 on the pain scale of 0 to 10. Once the patient rates their pain at 5 or higher, it's virtually impossible to reduce it. This is the key to pain management.

It's understandable that family members are often afraid of administering pain medication to their loved one. What if they do it wrong?

But when a doctor determines a diagnosis that states your loved one has six months or less to live, your loved one is generally sent home from a hospital and admitted to home hospice care. The hospice organization will then order a comfort kit that contains pain medications. Your hospice nurse can then train you how to administer these properly, and this is one of the most vital skills to learn for home hospice care. In chapter 3, you will also learn the nonverbal cues that let you know when someone is in pain. These can help if you are ever called upon to provide pain control to a loved one who can no longer communicate what they are feeling. This way, they don't have to be able to let you know when they need more medication to be comfortable.

It's important to note that palliative sedation is *legal everywhere in the US* and in many countries throughout the world. It is *not* euthanasia or physician-assisted suicide. When a patient needs more medication to ease their pain, however, some people view it as a version of slow euthanasia. But that is inaccurate. It is merely used to control symptoms, not to shorten someone's life.

Obviously, whenever possible, it's important to discuss the use of such medications with your loved one before the necessity to use them arises. When someone can make their wishes known, you can feel confident that you are abiding by what they want and helping them avoid unnecessary pain.

People will either die comfortably, or they will die suffering.

VOLUNTARILY STOPPING EATING AND DRINKING (VSED)

Phyllis Shacter had been happily married to Alan for twenty-six years. But then he was diagnosed with both Alzheimer's disease and laryngeal cancer. In a TEDx Talk and her book, *Choosing to Die*, Phyllis told the story of Alan's decision to end his life through VSED, which stands for voluntarily stopping eating and drinking.

While VSED is legal in all fifty US states for terminal patients to hasten their death, Alan had to make that choice while he was still mentally competent to do so. He decided it was time to implement it when he became too tired to take part in the activities he had always enjoyed. He fasted for nine and a half days, and as his body became dehydrated, he asked only for mists of water and some medication to keep him comfortable.

Phyllis watched him gradually go into a coma as his breathing quieted, and he died peacefully at home. As she put it, "There is a very important distinction to make between suicide and Alan's choice.... Suicide is about saying NO to life. Alan was saying YES to life, up to his last breath, on his terms."[4]

VSED usually causes death within seven to fourteen days, and it mimics the natural way the body dies. Some people find the extra time reassuring because it provides space for them to say goodbye to their loved ones. Most people don't find it uncomfortable to stop eating, but it's important to keep the patient's mouth moist and have medication available (see the previous section on palliative sedation) so that the dehydration doesn't cause discomfort. Most hospices condone VSED if the patient has set forth their wishes in writing while of sound mind, and patients don't have to get government or physician approval to do it.[5]

VSED certainly isn't recommended for everyone, however, especially those who are suffering a great deal. When that's the case, palliative sedation, which I discussed in the previous section, is the preferred option as someone nears the end of life.

If you are not in the US and your loved one is interested in VSED, research the laws and practices in your country, as acceptance of this method varies greatly.

MEDICAL AID IN DYING (MAID)

While medical aid in dying (MAID) is currently legally available in only ten US states plus Washington, DC, and a few other countries, there is a movement to make it law in more US states in the years to come. It's a medical practice in which a terminally ill, mentally capable adult may request a prescription from their doctor for medication to end their life. This medication is self-administered by the patient; it isn't given to them by anyone else. Unlike palliative sedation, it is indeed a form of self-induced euthanasia.

In the states where this is legal, the patient must meet all four

---

criteria: (1) a prognosis of six months or less to live, (2) mental capacity to make this decision, (3) being age eighteen or older, and (4) ability to self-ingest the medication with their own hands.

The movement for MAID is driven by a fear of pain and loss of control, but palliative sedation and VSED, which are already available in all fifty states in the US and many other parts of the world, address pain and loss of control without the need for self-induced euthanasia. If more people understood that palliative sedation and VSED are available and how they work, they would realize they already have everything they need *right now* for a peaceful and painless death. MAID is another option but not as necessary as people think.

DYING WITH DIGNITY

Most people want to die with dignity. It's important to distinguish, however, between the organization called Death with Dignity, which is fighting for MAID, and simply dying with dignity, which for most people means being comfortable without pain and suffering, knowing they are being cared for, and having as much control over their end-of-life choices as they can, especially when what they consider "quality of life" is no longer possible for them.

Planning ahead to make our desires known is the best way I know to control our end of life as much as possible. When our loved ones know what we want, they can ensure we get it when we can no longer speak for ourselves. To a great degree, that's what this entire book is about.

THE GROUNDBREAKING RESEARCH
INTO PSYCHEDELICS

Contrary to what some people think, psychedelic medications do not lead to addiction or dependency. A 2020 article in *Scientific American* reported the following: "Scientists are rediscovering what many see as the substances' astonishing therapeutic potential for a vast range of issues, from depression to drug addiction and acceptance of mortality."[6] A great deal of research was conducted on these substances in the 1950s and 1960s, but then they got an unfounded reputation as dangerous and were banned.

Psilocybin is one such substance that naturally occurs in some kinds of mushrooms, which is why it's colloquially called "magic mushrooms." It has a long history of use among Indigenous cultures for healing and ceremonies. Currently, in the US, it's still a Schedule I substance under the Controlled Substances Act, which means it's illegal except for research and supervised use in some cities and states that have decriminalized it. Psilocybin also remains illegal in most countries, with only a handful of them having legalized it. Hopefully, this will start to change.

The studies involving psilocybin's potential for therapeutic use in a controlled environment are certainly promising. For example, for the treatment of the acute fear of death, studies have found that one standard dose is enough to recalibrate how someone feels about dying.

Dr. Anthony P. Bossis of the New York University School of Medicine calls psilocybin and other psychedelic substances like it "meaning-making medicines." He outlined his research in a TEDx Talk called "Psychedelics and Psychology: Modern Medicine Meets

Ancient Medicine." He talked about dying patients who took psilocybin and described having feelings of wonder, awe, humility, gratitude, transcendence, and transformation. He said the drug provided them with a mystical experience and a strong sense of interconnectedness. One patient dying of cancer said, "Death doesn't matter." Another reported feeling that they weren't just their body or their illness. One woman felt completely encompassed by love, and even though she was an atheist, she felt she couldn't describe it any other way than God's love. As a result, these patients experienced dramatic reductions in anxiety and depression toward the end of their lives.[7]

Naturally, we can't prove that what people experience under the influence of psilocybin or other psychedelics is real, but we can't prove it isn't either. In the future, thanks to the research of scientists like Dr. Bossis, this experience may be available to more people who are suffering from an intense fear of death as they near the end of their life.

EASING OUR FEAR OF DEATH

In the past, observing the profound fear of death in most of my patients, their families, and the medical professionals around me, I believed there must be something incredibly terrible that awaits us after we die. What else could justify the desperate attempts to cling to life that I saw on a daily basis? Yet in my search for this awful truth, I found nothing of the sort. Many patients who were nearing the end of their lives shared beautiful experiences and visions similar to those described by the patients taking psilocybin.

Personally, I have never felt more alive than when I began working with individuals nearing death. It has given me a deep sense of gratitude that permeates every aspect of my existence. I will share these gifts with you as you continue reading these chapters, but one of them is the recognition that death is the ultimate equalizer of our shared humanity. No one is spared this reality regardless of their economic status or societal standing. No one can buy their way out of it. Whether we live in one of the world's largest cities or on a tiny island in the South Pacific, our body shuts down at the end of life in the same way. Therefore, death serves as a powerful reminder of the similarities that bind us together.

Of course, no one knows exactly what happens after we die, but the evidence based on what people at end of life have reported has caused me to lose my fear of death. You will hear a lot more about my experiences in this regard before you complete this book, but here's one for you.

A little girl named Tammy was about six years old when her grandmother was dying. Her grandma was everything to her. When it was time for the two of them to say goodbye, everyone left the room and allowed them some time alone. Tammy helped her grandma put on lipstick because that's one of the things they always did together. Then Grandma said to her, "Don't be afraid. It's beautiful!" She planted kisses all over Tammy's face, leaving behind red lipstick prints, and then gently died. When the others came back into the room, they were beside themselves with grief. But little Tammy stood there with those red lip prints on her face and told them, "Don't be afraid. She said it's beautiful!"

Are we missing out on the profound teachings that death holds for us by turning away from its presence? Perhaps it's time to reevaluate our relationship with death.

As you continue reading, you will learn more and more about what to expect when someone is nearing death. My hope is that your fears will dissipate with each page and that by the last page, you will feel much more peaceful about this inevitable transition we all share.

"MEANING CAN BE FOUND IN LIFE LITERALLY UP TO
THE LAST MOMENT, UP TO THE LAST BREATH,
IN THE FACE OF DEATH."
—*Viktor Frankl*

In the next chapter, we will talk about the options we have for preparing for end of life as our lifespans are now often longer than in the past.

2

Preparing for Longer Lifespans: The Elder Care Crisis

> Nothing in life is to be feared; it is only to be understood. Now is the time to understand more, so that we may fear less.
>
> —Marie Curie

When Marcia's mother had to go into a hospital, the doctors were clear: Her advanced Parkinson's disease had reached a point where she would need a live-in nurse or nursing home care. "My father was unwilling to have a nurse in his home, so even though he didn't want my mother in a nursing home either, we had little choice," Marcia says. She was left to scramble to find a nursing facility that would take her mother. This proved to be a difficult task.

"Most of the ones that had an available bed were too far away from where my parents lived. I needed a place close by so that my father could visit Mom easily. And time was of the essence," she recalls.

Marcia finally did find a nursing home, and her mother obtained Medicaid coverage. Since her parents hadn't done any estate planning, their house was still in both their names. Medicaid allowed her father to stay in the house, but then he died first. That left the house solely in her mother's name, which meant she was no longer eligible for Medicaid coverage.

"As my mother's legal guardian, I then had to pay directly for her nursing care, and the only funds I would have for that would be from the sale of their house," Marcia says. "But the court wanted to make sure I didn't run away with the funds, so they said I needed a bond before they would allow me to sell the house. As someone with few assets, I couldn't secure a bond, and for a while, it looked like I would have to relinquish guardianship of my mother to a stranger appointed by the court. It was utterly heartbreaking. I was lucky that a lawyer friend of mine was willing to cosign a bond for me, but even with that, he could only find one company willing to provide it. Thankfully, this allowed me to sell the house and pay for Mom's care from the proceeds. She lived another nine months, but I had to deal with all of this right after the death of my father. It was the most stressful experience of my life."

Unfortunately, what Marcia went through isn't uncommon. Most people don't put plans into place before their lives reach a crisis point. Then, everything becomes urgent, and they're left to make decisions while in a state of overwhelm. Sometimes, as in Marcia's case, our loved one is no longer able to make decisions for themselves. So we have to do it for them, hoping that we make the right ones since we've never talked to them about their wishes.

As our aging population is growing globally at an astounding rate, more and more people are going to be in this position. In fact, life expectancy has nearly doubled over the last century, and the longer we live, the more likely we are to experience physical, cognitive, and financial complications. For this reason, the senior population is becoming one of the largest demographics experiencing poverty.[1] You may have heard about the declining global birth rate and how it could impact the future of civilization. The main concern is that an overwhelming aging population and a much lower percentage of young people will likely cause strain on the labor market and the economy. In most parts of the world, we're entering a monumental demographic shift, as those aged sixty-five and older begin to out-number children and teens for the first time in history.

The World Health Organization estimates that by the year 2050, the number of people in the world who are sixty and older will dou-ble, and the number of people who are eighty and older will triple. According to Census.gov, from 1920 to 2020, the older population in the US grew from 4.9 million to 55.8 million. This is an alarming growth rate of about 1,000 percent, which is nearly five times higher than the growth of the total population at 200 percent. By the year 2030, about 23 percent of the US population will be sixty-five or older. It's an unprecedented time, and this shift is expected to con-tinue for decades.

Unfortunately, the United States and many other countries don't have the systems and infrastructure in place to care for their elder populations properly. The cost of everything continues to rise, and we simply aren't prepared to support people in health care, housing, or living as they age. We already saw how hospitals around the world quickly became overwhelmed during the Covid-19 pandemic. The elder care crisis is arriving more gradually, but the wave of people needing care is building up before we have enough hospital beds and medical personnel.

This is why we all need to take matters into our own hands as early as possible to make sure we are prepared *before* we find ourselves in a stressful state of crisis.

Unless we ask the right questions while our loved one is still well and of sound mind, we can't know what they would prefer. That's what this chapter is about: making decisions ahead of time and being as ready as possible for what might come.

LIVING WELL AGING PLANS

In the free Doulagivers Institute training, we recommend that people make three Living Well Aging Plans that we call A, B, and C. Later in the book, you will be directed to sit down with your loved one to formally write down all of these plans. This chapter and the ones that follow will provide vital information that you can refer back to when you create those plans.

Living Well Aging Plan A is the best-case scenario. Ask your loved one: If you had no physical or mental limitations and no money issues, where would you want to live? For example, maybe they want to live in New York City and attend theater on a regular basis. What financial considerations are necessary for that to happen?

Living Well Aging Plan B is if your loved one has some physical or mental limitations requiring some help, but they are primarily doing okay. For example, if they can no longer use the stairs, and the bathroom and bedroom are on the second floor, what options do they have? Can they install a bathroom and bedroom on the main floor? Can they move to a different location? Is there a family member with a first-floor bathroom and bedroom where they can live? Is assisted living an option?

Living Well Aging Plan C is your loved one's plan if they become completely incapacitated and unable to do anything for themselves. In other words, they need 24/7 care. Where would they like that care to take place? What housing and financial resources are available? Are there active family members around to support them? Are they eligible for services like Medicaid, Meals on Wheels, or others that offer rides to medical appointments and the grocery store? Are there community and religious organizations that might help?

Bear in mind that according to *Forbes Health* in 2023, the average private room in a US nursing home ranges from $9,000 to $15,000 per month, while assisted living facilities usually cost $4,000 to $5,000 per month. Some countries with universal health care provide nursing home care as well, but as populations age worldwide, it will become more and more difficult for these countries to afford the cost of so many in need.

If there will be money issues, what are the realistic options?

If a patient is in the US, where Medicaid is an option, it's important to note that before deciding on coverage, the Medicaid agency will look at the previous five years of their finances. They do this to check for large money transfers that were made in order to make someone appear eligible when they might not be. So a trust, for example, must have been set up before that five-year period. A Medicaid trust is a possibility to preserve some funds, but it requires a lawyer to set up.

Medicaid eligibility requires that the patient maintain only a small amount of money in their bank account. This varies from state to state, so check your state's specific rules, and check into what's available in your country if you're outside of the US.

The harsh reality is that depending on where and how long

someone lives, even a great deal of money might not be enough for Plan A. I worked with a family on creating a plan for someone with Alzheimer's disease in his family tree. They had a bit more than $5 million, so they thought they could care for him at home even if Alzheimer's struck when he was in his late sixties. But when I did the math for them for 24/7 care, they realized that $5 million would perhaps last for a decade at best. And most of us don't have $5 million stashed away, so we need to come up with alternative solutions. Certainly, nursing home care will bleed our assets completely in a short time. Once the assets are exhausted, we are left with Medicaid in the US.

We will talk about estate planning later in the book, but it's important to be aware of the realities and what's truly possible as our loved ones age and approach death.

ADVANCE DIRECTIVES: THE LIVING WILL

Advance directives are legal documents that set forth what someone wants to happen if they are unable to speak for themselves. They consist of two documents. The first is sometimes called a living will, which sets forth that certain measures should not be taken to prolong the patient's life if they are incapacitated. One of the measures that people often decide to decline is resuscitation if they stop breathing. This is specifically called a do not resuscitate (DNR) order. A request for VSED (voluntarily stopping eating and drinking) can be added to a living will for dementia patients like Alan, whom you read about in chapter 1. There are also special advance directives for dementia in which someone can request that nutrition be stopped when they reach certain conditions in their illness.

Don't assume, however, that any advance directive document automatically means "do not treat." It can express both what the patient wants and doesn't want. Even if someone wants no further curative treatment, they should always be given palliative care, which is care and treatment to keep them pain-free and comfortable by addressing their medical, social, and spiritual needs.

It's also true that a DNR will not prevent emergency medical professionals from resuscitating the patient when responding to an emergency call. Unless the person has an "out-of-hospital DNR order," emergency personnel (at least in the United States) are required by law to attempt CPR before transporting someone to a hospital.

Most US states have advance directive documents online, but almost all of them are vague. While most states don't require a particular form, they might have witnessing and notarizing requirements or other special signing formalities that should be followed. Even if your state does require a specific form, doctors should respect your clearly communicated treatment wishes in whatever form they have been written down.

Unfortunately, living wills aren't common around the world. Only a few countries, such as Denmark, Spain, and Portugal, have a formal living will registry. But even if your country doesn't have available documents, *write down your loved one's wishes.* If you worry that others in your family might dispute an informal document, make an audio recording of your loved one's wishes as a backup. Just make sure those wishes are *specific and extensive,* which means that even if you download a document online, it may be too vague in and of itself.

When I finally got my mother to show me her living will, it was so vague that my first thought was "You should get your money back from the lawyer." Other than "I want to be comfortable and have a do not resuscitate order at the end," it didn't tell me anything about how to support her choices. (You'll learn more about specifics to include in chapter 8.)

The specificity in your loved one's living will is for you to know their wishes, for the family to know their wishes, and for medical personnel to know their wishes. Nevertheless, in most places around the world, even if the document has been witnessed and notarized, it is still *not* legally binding. Yes, you read that correctly. As a result, even though your loved one's doctors *should* abide by them, they can often refuse to comply if they have an objection of conscience or consider the patient's wishes to be medically inappropriate. And the law is on the doctors' side.

The truth is that these documents were not created to protect the patient. They were created to protect the doctor if they *did* follow the patient's wishes. That way, the family couldn't sue. But if a doctor does not want to comply with someone's living will, they should transfer the patient to another health care provider who will honor the documents. The best-case scenario is to discuss wishes with health care providers well in advance so that you can confirm their willingness to comply.

If you can't ensure that doctors will abide by the living will, even if discussed ahead of time, what can you do? If you are in the US and your loved one has been diagnosed with a serious illness, you can complete what is called a POLST form, which stands for physician orders for life-sustaining treatment, and is also referred to by other terms, such as medical orders for life-sustaining treatment (MOLST), physician orders for scope of treatment (POST), or transportable physician orders for patient preferences (TPOPP). This form is valid in all fifty states. (Of course, if you're in a country other than the US, you will have to check to see what is available to you in terms of legally binding advance directives, as it varies from place to place.) This is indeed a legally binding document, but the downside is that you can't complete it far in advance before a serious diagnosis. However, if your loved one has already created advance directives that are not legally binding, you will have all of the information you need to transfer to the POLST form.

This form must be completed by a doctor and is a medical order that all medical professionals must follow by law. It sets forth that CPR will not be done, so it is a DNR. People can specify whether they want to go into a hospital if they are still breathing and have a pulse, as well as the treatments they want while there, including whether they want to go into the intensive care unit and be put on a breathing machine, if necessary. They can also specify whether they want a feeding tube if they can no longer eat by mouth and whether they want to receive antibiotics. Often printed on brightly colored paper to make it easy to see and find, the POLST is our secret weapon for making sure that our wishes are followed to the letter when we are at end of life. These forms should be kept in the patient's medical records as well as at home. If an ambulance is called, they will need these forms. Otherwise, EMTs will automatically take measures that might be against the patient's wishes. Again, without final wishes set forth, medical personnel are obligated by law to try to keep someone alive by any means necessary.

You might think it's enough to just have conversations with your loved one about their wishes, but if you don't have those wishes set down on paper, you and your relatives might remember the conversation differently. I have personally witnessed this. I knew a woman who had a severe stroke and never regained her functioning, but she didn't have a living will for her family. Her son and daughter remembered having a conversation with her about her wishes, but one of them recalled that she wanted to do everything to survive, while the other one swore that she wanted no extreme measures to keep her alive. When the doctor told them their mother would need a feeding tube to survive, they had no idea what to do. I've seen families broken apart by these kinds of disagreements. So the best strategy is to combine discussions with documentation.

Sadly, two-thirds of all US adults have no living will or other advance directives,[2] and with living wills unusual in so many parts of the world, the numbers are often even worse in other countries. This leaves families and doctors at a loss as to what patients would want. And while most people think advance directives only make sense for older people, younger people are even more at risk of being kept alive in a vegetative state, perhaps for years. None of us knows when we might be in an accident or have an illness that renders us incapacitated. So it's a good idea to be prepared regardless of our age.

Even older people sometimes feel uncertain or ambivalent about what they would want if incapacitated, so they put off creating their living will. But this is a recipe for ending up in worst-case scenarios. After all, we can always revise the document if we change our mind later.

While it's best to have a living will that communicates a patient's wishes, it isn't absolutely necessary in order to stop treatment near the end of life. Physicians generally consult with the family when the dying can't speak for themselves. The goal is for the family to make the decision the dying would make if they could.

Whatever advance directives are created, it's important not to be vague and to have answers ready for more than just whether or not we want resuscitation. I will provide the questions that need to be asked in part 2 of this book, "The Peace of Mind Planner."

ADVANCE DIRECTIVES: THE HEALTH CARE PROXY

The second part of advance directives is usually called a health care proxy document, although the name may vary depending on where you live. For example, it might be called health care surrogate, health care power of attorney, medical power of attorney, or health care agent.

This form allows the patient to decide who will speak for them if they aren't able to speak for themselves, either physically or cognitively. There are misconceptions about this role, however. Some people say, "I couldn't possibly make life and death decisions for my mother!" But this is exactly where a health care proxy comes in. When your loved one specifies their wishes if they're incapacitated, the person named as proxy doesn't have to make the decisions. They are just tasked with making the patient's wishes known to medical professionals. This is one of the reasons why it's so important to plan ahead. That way, no one has to make decisions for the patient and wonder if they're making the best ones.

Nevertheless, for some family members, it's still too much to think about telling medical professionals what their loved one wants. It isn't necessarily an easy job when you are in the midst of grief. Therefore, it's important not to take this decision lightly. The health care proxy needs to be the right person. They need to feel that they can truly do this job and advocate for the patient. They need to fully understand and agree with the patient's wishes so that there aren't any conflicts. If the patient wants a DNR, but the health care proxy is against having a DNR, there will be a big problem. So this person needs to be a strong, solid support to voice the patient's choices when it counts.

For this reason, a family member may not be the best choice for this role. The health care proxy does not have to be a relative. It can be a friend, lawyer, clergyperson, or any other trusted person. They simply need to be eighteen years of age or older and someone who is comfortable with the patient's choices. It's also best, of course, if they live close by so that they can go to the hospital when necessary to converse with doctors. If medical personnel can't reach the health care proxy quickly, it's a problem.

The health care proxy should also make sure that all of the patient's advance directives are entered into medical records when necessary, especially if the patient is transferred from one medical facility to another. The health care proxy can also access the patient's medical records and discharge doctors.

What's the difference between a health care proxy form and a power of attorney? A health care proxy is used only for medical decisions when someone has become incapacitated. Someone who has been given power of attorney can make decisions for other types of matters depending on what the power of attorney document specifies.

The bottom line is that everyone, regardless of age, needs to legally appoint someone they trust to voice their medical decisions if it becomes necessary. Note that when someone turns eighteen years of age in the US, due to the HIPAA (Health Insurance Portability and Accountability Act), they need to create a living will and health care proxy form if they want their parent(s) to be their advocate. Once they are eighteen, their parents no longer automatically have the right to access their medical records or see that their wishes are honored.

Living will and health care proxy forms vary by state, so when you go online to find these, be sure to choose based on the state where the patient has their legal residence. If they reside in more than one state, these forms have to be completed for both states. If there are no such forms in your country, you can create one using the United States models. While they won't be legally binding, you will still have your loved one's wishes set forth for yourself and the rest of the family, and your loved one's physician may be willing to honor the documents as well.

HOUSING SOLUTIONS

As I said, housing is often a big problem as we age. Most people say they would rather spend their last years at home, and the truth is that in the majority of cases, medical facilities aren't the most appropriate place for end of life. They are designed to focus on preventing diseases and providing cures. Since there is no cure for death, this isn't a viable, sustainable, or affordable way to provide end-of-life care (even if it's logistically possible). Considering the increasing elder population, we can assume that soon there won't be enough nursing facilities for the numbers of people who might be eligible for them—even if they can afford it.

End-of-life care is about providing the highest quality of daily life for the patient and their family. It's about planning for the inevitable so that it goes as well as possible, upholding the patient's wishes, maintaining their dignity, and making it easier for the family.

Whenever possible, I advocate bringing back the multigenerational family unit and potentially sharing the care of our elders. For example, one family member might take the elder person for six months and another for the next six months. This prevents anyone from burning out physically, emotionally, or financially.

There are also "granny pods" (sometimes called accessory dwelling units or ADUs), which are a modern-day solution to a modern-day problem. These are small, detached guest houses that can be placed in a backyard. Similar to an in-law cottage or mother-in-law suite, they are one level with a bedroom, bathroom, living area, and kitchenette. This is especially helpful if no one in the family has a home with a ground-floor bathroom or bedroom.

These pods come in all types of designs from nautical to log cabin, and they can be equipped with safety features like ankle-level cameras, hand railings, slip-resistant floors, wide doorways, rounded countertops, soft floors, lighted floorboards, oxygen, and voice-activated emergency communication systems. You can know, for example, when your loved one's feet land on the floor each morning and keep tabs on them while allowing them some independence and the family some privacy.

These pods are usually hooked up to the sewer, water, and power lines of the main house, but regulations and zoning laws vary depending on where you live. So you'll have to check the rules to make sure you're in compliance.

The cost of granny pods varies based on factors like location, size, and features, but on average in the US, they range from $70,000 to

$250,000. You can buy a kit or a prefabricated version. The prices may sound expensive, but when you compare them to the cost of assisted living facilities, they become quite affordable.

One of my visions with Doulagivers that is just beginning to come to fruition is the development of Doula Communities with Doula Houses. These will be holistic communities and homes for the elderly, especially for people who don't have children or family. Our first of these communities is currently being developed in the country of Belize. Unfortunately, the bureaucracy in the US is complicated, so it's currently easier to make them happen in other countries. But I'm hopeful that we will be able to create them in the US before long.

SOLUTIONS EXIST

As you can see, even though the outlook seems stark for us as we age and outgrow the younger population, there are potential solutions that can make it easier, the first of which is planning ahead! I can't reiterate enough how important it is to not only help our loved ones plan for their end of life but to plan for our own, no matter how old we are.

Exercise: Create Living Well Aging Plans
In this chapter, you have learned the basics of Living Well Aging Plans. It's now time to help your loved one create theirs in writing (and perhaps go ahead and create your own). If you're working with someone else to develop their plans, discuss their options carefully. You may need to do some research on such things as their finances, available nursing homes, and Medicaid eligibility.

Remember that **Living Well Aging Plan A** is the best-case scenario. If they had no physical or mental limitations and no money issues, where would they want to live? If there aren't currently enough funds for this option, is there enough time to gather them?

For **Living Well Aging Plan B**, talk about where they would live if they had some physical or mental limitations. Speak to family about possibly sharing responsibility, and think about first-floor bathrooms and bedrooms if stairs are no longer an option. Is a granny pod or assisted living facility a possibility?

For **Living Well Aging Plan C**, look at the housing and financial resources that are available to your loved one if they become completely incapacitated. Would 24/7 home care be possible, and are there family members available to provide some or all of this care? If not, research nursing homes now to determine which ones would be best. Even though circumstances could change, it's still a good idea to find out if your loved one would likely be accepted at the top nursing homes of choice. Conduct research to determine eligibility for services such as the ones we have in the US, like Medicaid, Meals on Wheels, or other services that offer rides to medical appointments and the grocery store. Look into community and religious organizations that might help.

You will work with these plans further when creating the Financial Good Death Peace of Mind Plan in chapter 11.

In the next chapter, we'll talk about the three phases of end of life and why it's important to understand them and plan for them.

3

How to Care for Someone Who Is Dying: The Three Phases of End of Life

The greatest tribute to the dead is not grief but gratitude.

—Thornton Wilder

One beautiful spring day in the Hudson Valley, I drove my trusty Honda Civic along the winding country back roads to meet a new hospice patient for the first time. Her name was Christine, and she'd moved to live with her son, Michael, and his family after she was diagnosed with a terminal illness. I drove through miles and miles of rolling hillsides and lush vegetation in majestic colors. It was so moving to be surrounded by such natural beauty while on my way to care for a dying human being.

As I pulled into the dirt driveway, I saw their wooden cabin-like house perched at the top of the hill. The setting was so peaceful... until Michael answered the door. He was shaking visibly as he held a syringe of medication in his hand.

"What's going on here?" I asked myself as I followed him into the kitchen. I was grateful I had a good poker face, because I certainly didn't want to add to his anxiety.

After some questioning, I found out that the doctor who discharged Christine from the hospital made a comment to Michael that his mother was at risk of a blood clot breaking off in her lungs, causing her to die of suffocation. He'd been told that the only thing that could possibly help with that situation would be liquid morphine—hence the syringe in his hand when I arrived. But nothing in Christine's medical history or disease process supported the conclusion that she was at high risk for blowing a blood clot. Nevertheless, the doctor's comment had scared the daylights out of Michael. He believed he needed to be ready at any moment and was worried he wouldn't be able to do right by his mother.

Michael and his family were clearly in the first of three distinct phases that we all go through when someone is at the end of life:

1. Shock
2. Stabilization
3. Transition

When we're aware of each of these phases, we can prepare for them, put a plan in place, and understand that what we're experiencing is a natural part of the process. We can know what to expect and more easily calm ourselves and others down as we move through each aspect of the end of life. In my experience, death can be a sacred, beautiful experience when we're educated about each of these phases and the best way to handle them. Let's take a look at each one.

THE SHOCK PHASE

When I arrived at their house, Michael and his family were deep in the throes of the shock phase, which occurs right after someone has received a terminal diagnosis. Learning that Christine was on the verge of death had turned their whole world upside down, and they were experiencing a host of understandable emotions from fear and depression to anger and denial.

I recognized this phase immediately, and thankfully, I was in a position to relieve at least a little bit of Michael's angst by letting him know he needn't worry so much about blood clots or his ability to administer morphine to his mother at that time. (There would be time to teach him how to do it later, when his mother would need it.) Then I proceeded to teach him what I teach all caregivers in this situation.

In order to help a loved one who is facing the shock of their diagnosis, the most important thing you can do at first is *listen*. Remember that whatever you're experiencing, they've just learned their time left is limited, and they need space to process and grieve as much as you do, perhaps even more so. Don't try to talk them out of their feelings or pretend the reality is different from what it is. Simply *be present* for them to the best of your ability, and allow them to express their shock, fear, anger, depression, and pain. *Don't judge.* Meet them where they are emotionally, and accept whatever they feel and say. Your nonjudgmental presence is the best possible salve, and it will build trust with them so that they will feel comfortable expressing more and deeper feelings with you. As they talk, just nod to convey your understanding. If you say anything, you might want to say, "I understand" or "I get it." You're validating whatever they feel without trying to get them to feel something different.

When anyone is given a terminal diagnosis, they feel utterly out of control. One of the ways you can give them back some control is by asking, "What can I do for you? Do you have any immediate needs?" Pain and discomfort are in the category of "immediate needs." Of course, you might have to check with medical professionals about what to do for some of these issues, but you might be able to take care of others right away, such as adjusting a pillow or providing a glass of water. You're aiming for the highest quality of life every day.

It's important to continue to ask this question every day or perhaps even more than once per day until the end. When someone is nearing the end of life, their immediate needs can change quickly.

Also, check for safety issues. At some point, your loved one may no longer be able to stand up and walk or even to swallow. So it's important to watch for these signs, especially if you're still in the midst of the shock phase, as these issues can show up at any time. I can't count the number of times a patient broke their hip or some other bone because they got up and tried to go to the bathroom when they weren't able to walk anymore. So safety issues are major, and we need to prepare for them, making sure support is always present to prevent accidents if at all possible.

This also means that as the caregiver—just like Michael, who was the main caregiver for Christine—you are embroiled in your own shock and the host of emotions that accompany it. Therefore, it's vital to be gentle with yourself, as well as to take care of yourself physically and emotionally while you process your new reality. You can't expect yourself to be present at all times to mitigate safety issues and take care of the dying person's needs.

There's something we call "caregiver syndrome," where someone taking on the brunt of the responsibility for the dying person burns out, becomes physically ill, or reaches their emotional limit (we will discuss this further in chapter 5). I work with my clients to create a rotating support system with others in the family or friendship circle so that everything doesn't fall on one person's shoulders. Do whatever possible to receive the support *you* need during this time as well. Only through taking care of yourself can you truly be present and beneficial to your dying loved one. You will require breaks and periods of respite.

No matter how well you navigate through this time, it isn't easy. So give yourself moments to sit with your own feelings, and remember to check in with yourself regularly. Be willing to ask others for what you need.

To review, these are the main interventions during the shock phase:

1. Build trust by being fully present and listening.
2. Meet people where they are emotionally without judgment.
3. Give them back some control by asking, "What can I do for you?" and checking for safety issues.

THE STABILIZATION PHASE

Stabilization occurs when the dying person's pain is hopefully under control, they're still lucid and able to express themselves, and all acute issues that were identified during the shock phase have been adequately addressed. This leads to the highest quality of daily living for everyone involved. When things are stable, the shock is finally over, and there's a window of opportunity to have important conversations and say goodbyes. Wonderful work can be done during this phase to make the death less emotionally painful for everyone involved. This is the perfect time to say what we want to say, so there's nothing left unsaid.

If your loved one hasn't made their wishes known yet, the stabilization phase is an excellent time to bring this up. Ask them what they would like, such as a particular type of music to be played or perhaps an aromatherapy scent that they love. Once I had a patient ask to hear a Bee Gees live album on rotation, so we ended up playing it for seventy-four hours straight!

Here are a few ways to create a beautiful, loving space for the dying person:

- Soft background music
- Dim lighting/candles
- Light aromatherapy (lavender scent or whatever the person desires)
- Gentle touch. The most comforting thing for the dying person is to know that someone is there taking care of them.
- Pets. Allow these unconditionally loving beings to be present to snuggle or lie next to their loved one at the end of life. They bring incredible comfort, and they also deserve to have this time with their human.

You will make notes of all of these and more when you get to the Peace of Mind Planner later in the book.

The stabilization phase is also the perfect time to ask the dying person questions about their life and allow them to reflect in what we often call a "life review," in which they can share beautiful insights from their journey and recount the contributions they made to the world. At the end of life, an organic moment often opens up for people to look back at their life from a different perspective. They frequently see experiences that caused them pain, shame, or anger with new clarity and without judgment. I have heard many people say, "I finally understand why that happened to me." They see that every experience in life, even the negative ones, is an opportunity to learn and grow as a human being. As they go over their life story, listen and validate their feelings.

It's also the best time to encourage family members to have one-on-one visits with the person who is on the verge of dying. Allow for private conversations, as long as the dying person is okay with these. Special goodbyes and the opportunity to say "I love you" are vital for reaching peace and acceptance, both for the dying and for those left behind. (I'll give you some guidelines for this in the book's Peace of Mind Planner.)

I once worked with a family whose patriarch was in hospice. I sat at the kitchen table with his wife and adult son, who was forty-seven and a tall man at six feet, five inches. While we reviewed what to expect as the man of the house was entering his last days, the son suddenly stood and pushed the table away with force. "So we're just going to give up then?" he said angrily, and stormed out of the house.

Just two days later, the son walked out of his father's bedroom with tears streaming down his cheeks. "Dad told me he loved me," he said calmly and peacefully. I felt as though I was looking at a six-year-old boy in a grown man's body. I didn't ask, but I suspected it was the first time he had ever heard those words from his father.

The stabilization phase is a good time as well to deal with unresolved issues, which can prevent people from having a good, peaceful death. These issues can also make grief more complicated for those who are left, and these conversations can allow for forgiveness. The dying person may want to talk about regrets, but only if everyone involved can approach the conversation with love. This isn't the time for anger and blame. It's the time for closure and letting go of grievances as best we can.

Throughout my career as a hospice nurse and Doulagiver, I have seen forgiveness consistently be one of the biggest factors that brings about a good death, and there is no better time for that than during the stabilization phase. Releasing heavy negative emotions can have a dramatic impact on our lives and allow us to heal. Forgiveness is the path to unconditional love. It's the intentional act of letting go of something that no longer serves us.

It's important to acknowledge, however, that forgiveness doesn't mean forgetting or condoning offenses. It doesn't mean we absolve someone for what they did. Forgiveness is for *us,* not the offender. If we can offer forgiveness to a loved one who is dying, that's wonderful, but the most important part of the process is to set ourselves free from our grievances.

If you aren't sure what to say, you might choose to simply say the following, which allows for letting go of the past and expressing what most needs to be said:

I forgive you.
Please forgive me.
Thank you.
I love you.

To review, these are the main interventions in the stabilization phase:

1. Do a life review with your dying loved one.
2. Encourage family members to have alone time with the dying person.
3. Practice forgiveness.

THE TRANSITION PHASE

The transition phase is the time right before a person dies. It marks the transition from this world into the next and can last anywhere from hours to days. As the dying person's body begins to shut down, it goes through fast changes that can make this phase particularly stressful.

Some people wait to die until they reach a certain milestone or until they can see a particular loved one. (We'll discuss this in more detail in the Epilogue.) If this is the case, try to facilitate a meeting with the person they may want to see, remain calm, create as sacred a space as possible (we'll discuss that in the Peace of Mind Planner as well), and work through your own emotions as best you can.

To assist someone in having a good death, you also need to understand the common indicators that they're entering this phase:

- Loss of the desire to eat or the ability to swallow food
- Agitation or restlessness. Sometimes they talk about having to "go home" or go on a trip somewhere.
- Sleeping most of the time or a sleeping coma. When

this happens, you can consider making them more comfortable by turning and positioning them with padding on any bony areas of their body.

- Incontinence
- Confusion and/or hallucinations
- Breathing changes, such as shallow breathing or periods of apnea, where they may seem to be breathing less frequently. Or they may do the opposite and go into a period of rapid breathing. At this point, you might ask the caregiver/nurse to administer a liquid morphine–Ativan mixture inside their cheek/mouth to provide comfort.
- A considerable increase or decrease in their body temperature. If they're cold, layer warm blankets over them. If they have a high temperature, put a cool wet cloth on their forehead and/or give them a Tylenol suppository.
- Skin color changes, usually paleness and possibly bluish lips and nails. The skin on their arms and legs may also look mottled. If this happens, try to keep them warm. If their hands and feet are cold, you can try gently rubbing them in your hands.
- Gurgling noises in the chest. Try adjusting the head of the bed to a forty-five-degree angle, if possible, or fold a pillow in half lengthwise and put it behind their back so that they can turn on their side. This will dislodge the secretions in the chest, which will hopefully cause the gurgling to stop.

To review, these are the main interventions of the transition phase:

1. Understand all the natural signs of this phase.
2. Make the dying person as comfortable as possible.
3. Note if there are any reasons they might be waiting to die.

THE IMPORTANCE OF SYMPTOM MANAGEMENT AND COMFORT TRACKING

If you track your loved one's symptoms, you can provide the highest quality of daily living every day throughout all three of the phases. This is the goal of end-of-life care.

As a hospice nurse, I identified the five categories that family caregivers need to assess every day. When you do, it will ensure that any issues are identified and managed quickly.

The tracker allows whoever is taking care of your loved one in the moment to make note of symptoms, so when you aren't around, you will still be able to monitor them. Then, when your hospice nurse comes to visit, or your loved one sees a physician, you will have an accurate, detailed, and concise record of pain, sleep, and more. Plus, the next time a doctor asks, "How have they been sleeping over the last month?" you'll have much more than a vague answer based on your best recollection. You will be able to answer any questions about your loved one's symptoms.

The tracker allows you to monitor for the following five categories:

Pain management. Monitor your loved one's pain level and response to the prescribed pain medication several times a day, as pain at the end of life can increase quickly. Therefore, the pain dosage that currently works well may not be adequate for good pain control in the future. Tight pain assessment and management is key to keeping your loved one comfortable throughout their entire end-of-life process.

Administer the medication as prescribed, and assess the effectiveness by asking your loved one thirty to forty-five minutes after they took the medication to rate their pain on a scale of 0 to 10. Their pain should be 4 or below. Remember that when the pain level reaches 5 or above, it's very difficult to bring it down. So it's vital to stay ahead of the pain for pain management!

Communicate with the hospice team or health care provider if the dosage needs to be adjusted based on the pain assessment. This is one of the greatest supports you can provide. (If your loved one is unable to communicate their pain level, later in the chapter, I will explain some nonverbal pain cues for you to use to assess their pain.)

People sometimes worry that pain medication will prevent their loved one from communicating, but that isn't usually the case until the very end of life, when the pain might be at its most intense. If someone complains of pain that's at a level of 4, they will be thrilled to bring it down to 1 or 2, which should allow them to remain communicative.

Nausea. This can rival pain and is present in many people at end of life, especially if they've recently had chemotherapy. Nausea travels via three different pathways in the brain, so it's crucial to have a compound antiemetic medication available for your loved one. The hospice comfort kit you receive should include one, but if not, ask for it. Then make sure to ask your hospice nurse to instruct you on when and how to administer it.

Sleep. Your loved one will require more and more sleep as their body becomes weaker. Make sure to give them ample downtime. Stagger visits with friends and family, and keep the visits short when necessary. Remember that even time with a dear friend can require lots of energy from someone who is dying. Give your loved one control by asking them when they want visits and with whom.

Each day, write down how many hours of sleep they received and the quality. You can ask them in the morning to let you know how well they slept on a comfort scale from 0 to 10, with 0 as fully comfortable and 10 as most uncomfortable.

Eating. People at the end of life don't require a lot of food. It's best to offer small, frequent meals that are of soft consistency, such as yogurt, ice cream, and pureed foods. Don't pressure, guilt, or force food on them. Just offer.

Remember that one of the first telltale signs that someone is heading into their transition phase is that they stop eating and drinking. This is an expected part of the process, but it can be alarming to families when they don't know about it. It's a natural way that the body starts to shut down. This is the time to provide maximum comfort with mouth swabs and mouth lubricants. You can repeat this care every few hours as needed.

Bowel movements. It's very important to monitor your loved one's bowel movements. There are three factors at end of life that contribute to the high probability of constipation: decreased mobility, decreased fluid intake, and use of narcotic medications. Constipation can bring great discomfort, but it can also become an emergency situation if impaction (blockage) occurs.

Your loved one should be having a bowel movement every one to two days. So if constipation is an issue, make sure there is a gentle laxative and stool softener on their medication list. If there is no bowel movement for more than two days, call your hospice nurse or medical provider.

NONVERBAL PAIN CUES

When someone is suffering but unable to ask for interventions to alleviate their pain, they will often provide nonverbal cues that let their caregivers know they are in pain. The following list shows the main cues you might notice if someone needs to increase their pain medication while in a sleeping coma.

Before they reach the sleeping coma stage, however, you can assure them that you know the nonverbal cues to look for if they are in pain, and that you will monitor them for these cues and do everything you can to prevent them from suffering. If any of these cues is fleeting, it may have been the result of a quick moment of pain or a dream that doesn't necessitate additional medication, but if the cues are sustained, consider them a sign of pain.

- Grimacing
- Pursed lips
- Furrowed eyebrows
- Wrinkled nose
- Tightly closed eyes
- Moaning or crying
- Tightened jaw
- Grinding teeth
- Clenched fists
- Rapid pulse
- Flinching
- Fidgeting or restlessness
- Rapid or labored breathing
- Tense or rigid muscles
- Clutching or guarding a specific part of the body

DOULAGIVERS END-OF-LIFE
SYMPTOM MANAGEMENT COMFORT TRACKER

DATE AND TIME	PAIN MANAGEMENT rate pain 0-10	NAUSEA MANAGEMENT note incidence and any medication given	SLEEP ideally 6-8 hours; rate quality 0-10	EATING ideally 2-3 small meals	BOWEL MOVEMENTS ideally every 1-2 days	NOTES
Monday, Date: Time:						
Tuesday, Date: Time:						
Wednesday, Date: Time:						
Thursday, Date: Time:						
Friday, Date: Time:						
Saturday, Date: Time:						
Sunday, Date: Time:						

Using the Symptom Management Comfort Tracker

Every day, go to the tracker and answer the five daily categories. If you note anything that's out of the "comfort" range—anything that scores 4 or above (except for eating)—contact your hospice nurse. They don't know there's an issue unless you notify them, so don't hesitate to call!

Add the date and time of occurrence, as well as the scale of the symptom from 0 to 10 (where applicable, with 10 denoting the worst). Also, make notes about what's happening, how it was managed, and any next steps. To download a printable version of the example tracker below, visit Doulagivers.com/comfort-tracker.

KNOWLEDGE OF THE THREE PHASES
HELPS FACILITATE A GOOD DEATH

We only have one opportunity for the end of someone's life to go well. We can't go back and do it over. Understanding the three phases, along with how to perform tight symptom management, allows you to confidently care for someone at end of life. This knowledge can make for not only a good death, but a beautiful, peaceful, moving, and even life-affirming one.

Michael, the man in the chapter's opening story, who was terrified with the morphine syringe in his hand the day I met him, was finally able to enjoy wonderful celebrations with his mother while she was in the stabilization phase. He will cherish those moments with her for the rest of his life.

One day, when I was wrapping up a weekly visit at his house, he confided in me that his father had died while he was in college. He wasn't able to handle it at that young age, and it caused him to avoid his family and the entire situation. For twenty years, he had been living with heavy guilt about the way he acted then. He looked me in the eye and said, "I want to get this right with my mom." Not only did he "get it right," but his mother's death was one of the most profound end-of-life journeys I have ever witnessed.

I arrived at their house just a few hours after Christine had died. Michael and his wife answered the door with smiles on their faces. They were so excited. "We haven't touched her," they said. "You just have to see her." They said it with such love.

They had awakened around 6:00 a.m. and walked into Christine's bedroom to find her motionless, sitting up in bed with a smile on her face. She looked so serene and absolutely beautiful there in her white gown. I held my heart at the sight of her, knowing that she had truly experienced a good death. They gave me a pair of her pearl earrings as thanks, and they're still among my most cherished possessions.

Christine's death was a natural and even positive experience for them. Yes, they would miss her. Yes, they were sad to lose her. But she had to go, and because they knew what to do for her and everyone else involved during each of the three phases, her transition was the epitome of a good death for them all.

Now that you know about the three phases and how to manage symptoms, let's review what to expect with some of the most common diseases at end of life.

4

Dealing with Common Diseases at End of Life

> We will do all we can not only to help you die
> peacefully, but also to live until you die.
> —Cicely Saunders

t's a common misconception among some medical staff that the specific disease doesn't matter once a patient is receiving hospice care. But that just isn't true. The disease process significantly affects the interventions needed for comfort and quality of life. While the very final days may look similar regardless of the illness, the period leading up to those days varies greatly.

So if you're caring for your loved one at the end of life, understanding their unique disease process, its progression, and what to do to ensure their comfort can be the key to helping them have a good death. After reading, you will know the most important symptoms to look for and how to manage them. I call these tips "Doulagivers' pearls."

One thing that's true regardless of the particular disease is the importance of having morphine, Ativan, and a compound antiemetic medication in the home. Most hospice kits given to families contain these medications, but some don't. If they're missing from yours, be sure to ask for them. Morphine is, of course, to manage pain and shortness of breath; Ativan is to manage anxiety; and anti-emetic medication is for nausea/vomiting.

I worked with a woman who had chronic obstructive pulmonary disease (COPD), which you'll read about in a moment. She'd had several episodes of being unable to breathe, and her family called the emergency number (911 in the United States) several times, taking her back to the hospital each time, even though they could do no more for her in that situation than her family could do at home. In fact, getting an increased dose of morphine to ease the breathing or pain and discomfort can take hours in the hospital, while it can be ready to go at home in a matter of minutes.

Finally, the woman with COPD said to me, "I don't care if I can't breathe. You have to promise me that they won't call 911 and take me back to the hospital." I explained to her that if we gave her a slightly higher dose of morphine, it would put her in a sleep coma and keep her comfortable despite the shortness of breath.

I discussed this with her daughters to make sure they understood what to do the next time their mother struggled for breath. I explained that she would be going into a palliative coma with the next increase of morphine and would no longer be able to talk with them. I suggested they take the time before the increase in morphine to say everything to her they wanted to say. That way, they would have no regrets—nothing left unsaid.

When someone's death is inevitable, they will either die comfortably and peacefully or they'll die suffering. This chapter is all about making sure that anyone on your watch dies comfortably and peacefully. I will review some of the most common diseases we see at end of life and what you need to know as a caregiver in order to facilitate a good death.

We know that time is not on our side at the end of life. As difficult as this may seem, knowing the truth about what to expect will allow you to feel empowered and have what you need in place (in terms of both education and medication) to support your loved one. It's one of the most important things we are ever asked to do.

BE PREPARED

First, here are some general guidelines that are true of all of the disease processes.

1. Have liquid morphine, Ativan, and nausea medication in the home, and make sure the hospice nurse has taught you how to administer them and how to understand the dosage.
2. Pace your loved one's activities to avoid exhaustion.
3. Use all means to make your loved one's life easier. Some of these include a bedside toilet, small meals of soft food (even eating can make some people short of breath), and a bedside table to place important items within reach.
4. Make safety paramount. If your loved one is struggling to walk or has balance issues, they shouldn't be walking without assistance from another person or a walker. Remove any rugs or anything that might cause falls.

5. Before feeding your loved one, evaluate their ability to swallow, and stop immediately if they struggle. If they swallow improperly, it can lead to aspiration pneumonia.

6. Have conversations where family/friends do the talking and don't require your loved one to talk in long sentences.

7. Prepare visitors for how your loved one looks. It's best for people who are dying if their visitors don't visibly show their shock or repulsion at how the dying person looks or smells.

8. Keep visits short, and give control back to your loved one by letting them decide when someone visits and for how long.

9. Have a drill for what everyone will do in case of an acute episode. This can prevent unnecessary and stressful emergency calls.

10. Consider incorporating massage, acupuncture, Reiki, or other relaxation techniques to help alleviate discomfort.

11. Use medical equipment, when necessary, for safety and preserving energy. For example, this might mean a wheelchair, a walker, or a Hoyer lift, which allows someone to be lifted while their bed is changed and cleaned or lifted to be transferred somewhere else.

12. Consider counseling for the patient and the family to address fears, anxiety, and depression.

13. Provide a compassionate presence, allowing your loved one to share their thoughts and feelings without judgment.
14. Encourage conversations about meaning, hope, and legacy.
15. Facilitate connections with spiritual or religious services according to your loved one's beliefs and wishes (even if they don't align with your own).
16. Create a calm, controlled, stress-free environment.

THREE QUESTIONS TO ASK

1. What are the acute issues, such as pain or difficulty breathing?
2. Are there safety issues that need to be addressed?
3. Who makes up your support system? Who can you call when you need advice or assistance?

END-STAGE LIVER DISEASE

Liver disease is a case in point as to why understanding the specific disease process matters. While most people know the liver is a vital organ, few realize that liver disease often leads to breathing problems. Eventually, fluid called *ascites* begins to accumulate in the abdomen. When that happens, medical practitioners drain or "tap" the fluid. A medical procedure will attach a tube to the patient's abdomen and the nurse will teach the family how to drain it every day.

But as the person's end of life draws closer, there comes a point when the draining doesn't work anymore. There's just too much fluid, and within twenty-four to forty-eight hours, that fluid will start to obstruct breathing and can lead to suffocation.

While I was a hospice nurse, I visited a woman whose husband was dying of liver disease. The draining/tapping was no longer working, and I knew her husband was going to suffocate and die within two days at the most. His wife had no idea because no one had told her. It was awful. For this reason, I think liver disease is one of the most difficult of them all.

Tight symptom management is so important with this disease to make sure the patient doesn't suffer. When the fluid starts to build up and leads to shortness of breath, we need to be able to give our loved one more liquid morphine to put them in a palliative coma.

The liver is critical for filtering toxins, aiding digestion, and regulating blood clotting and other vital processes. When it fails, these systems deteriorate, and eventually lead to end-of-life diseases such as liver cancer, cirrhosis, liver failure, or hepatitis C.

SYMPTOMS OF END-STAGE LIVER DISEASE
1. Jaundice, which causes yellowing of the skin and eyes
2. Fatigue
3. Muscle wasting
4. Weight loss
5. Fluid accumulation in the stomach
6. Itchy skin that often feels like it's happening below the top layer of skin
7. Altered cognitive abilities due to high ammonia levels
8. Dilated blood vessels in the esophagus and stomach that can rupture

9. Pain
10. Anxiety from feelings of suffocation
11. Rapid respiratory rate as the body tries to get more oxygen
12. Increased pulse rate from the heart trying to get more oxygen into the body

WHAT TO DO TO EASE YOUR LOVED ONE'S PAIN AND DISCOMFORT (BESIDES THE GENERAL GUIDELINES AT THE BEGINNING OF THE CHAPTER)

1. Use liquid morphine and Ativan for pain management and shortness of breath.
2. Use supplemental oxygen for shortness of breath.
3. Be prepared with a cool cloth and hypoallergenic lotion for itchy skin.

CHRONIC OBSTRUCTIVE PULMONARY DISEASE (COPD)/EMPHYSEMA

COPD is a progressive disease that typically worsens over time and is caused by long-term exposure to irritants like cigarette smoke, air pollution, chemical fumes, or dust. COPD makes it hard to get air in through the airways and into and out of the lungs. There are two main types of COPD: (1) chronic bronchitis, or inflammation of the lungs, and (2) emphysema, or destruction of the lung tissue (so oxygen can't get into the body).

SYMPTOMS OF COPD/EMPHYSEMA

1. Shortness of breath (the main and most debilitating symptom)
2. Anxiety from feelings of suffocation
3. Rapid respiratory rate as the body tries to get more oxygen
4. Increased pulse rate from the heart trying to get more oxygen into the body
5. Shaking/trembling in the late stages from retaining too much carbon dioxide

WHAT TO DO TO EASE YOUR LOVED ONE'S PAIN AND DISCOMFORT (BESIDES THE GENERAL GUIDELINES AT THE BEGINNING OF THE CHAPTER)

1. Use liquid morphine and Ativan for pain management and shortness of breath.
2. Use supplemental oxygen for shortness of breath.
3. Don't subject the patient to secondhand smoke or other intense odors of any kind.

LUNG CANCER

I witnessed a death from lung cancer that was one of the most beautiful transitions I've ever seen. The dying woman, Donna, was only in her sixties. You could tell she hadn't had an easy life, but she was very fiery and smart. Her daughter, Phoebe, was in her early twenties and had a full head of dark brown curls. She had also inherited her mother's wonderful sass. I could tell they had a close relationship.

As I entered Donna's hospital room, the nurses were calling for more morphine, and I could tell that my patient was actively transitioning to death. She was in a sleep coma, and there were four family members surrounding her bed. Everyone was silent, and her daughter was in bed with her, cradling and rocking her. It looked as though her daughter was "birthing" her into the next world. It was heartbreaking and breathtaking at the same time.

While lung cancer is a terrible disease, it's often one of the most gentle death processes I've experienced. Since it affects breathing, it can lead to shortness of breath, but surprisingly, it usually doesn't. The most prevalent symptom as it progresses is typically a feeling of weakness.

Of course, it's a type of cancer that begins in the lungs, which are the two spongy organs in the chest responsible for breathing. It's also one of the most common and serious types of cancer, leading to a significant number of deaths worldwide each year. There are three main types, but the symptoms and interventions remain the same for all three.

SYMPTOMS OF END-STAGE LUNG CANCER
1. Persistent cough
2. Coughing up blood
3. Pain in the ribs
4. Wheezing
5. Weakness (often the biggest complaint)
6. Shortness of breath

WHAT TO DO TO EASE YOUR LOVED ONE'S PAIN AND DISCOMFORT (BESIDES THE GENERAL GUIDELINES AT THE BEGINNING OF THE CHAPTER)

1. Administer small doses of liquid morphine for persistent cough, shortness of breath, or pain.
2. Use ibuprofen when there is a diagnosis of bone pain, which can develop in late stages. An anti-inflammatory drug works in this case, while a narcotic such as morphine does not work.
3. Pace activities to relieve shortness of breath and weakness.
4. Use supplemental oxygen.

PANCREATIC CANCER

Pancreatic cancer is a type of cancer that begins in the tissues of the pancreas, an organ in the abdomen that lies horizontally behind the lower part of our stomach. It plays an essential role in digestion by producing enzymes that the body needs to digest fats, carbohydrates, and proteins. It also produces hormones that help manage blood sugar levels, which are crucial for energy.

Unfortunately, pancreatic cancer has no early symptoms, so in most cases by the time it has been found, it's already in the late stages and fatal. It causes significant pain and moves quickly. Younger people in their forties, fifties, and sixties sometimes get it, and the life expectancy after diagnosis is often no more than three months. For this reason, it's hard for patients and their loved ones to have enough time to move out of the shock phase.

That's what it was like for Maggie, a patient of mine who had also been a nurse. She was only in her forties, and she had three daughters who were all in their early twenties. When I first arrived at Maggie's home, I was surprised to find her all alone. It was clear that her husband and her daughters were still in such shock that they were in denial about what was happening. Meanwhile, Maggie was in a lot of pain and experiencing extreme nausea. She was also struggling to walk, trying to stabilize herself by holding on to the wall. This was not safe! She had also resisted pain medications because she was worried they would make her constipated.

I talked with her about taking both pain medications and laxatives, if necessary. I didn't want her to endure pain unnecessarily just because of this fear. I also spoke to her family, letting them know that it was time for them to take leave from work to be with Maggie, have important conversations with her while they could, and make sure she received the care she needed.

SYMPTOMS OF PANCREATIC CANCER

1. Pain
2. Nausea (sometimes worse than the pain)
3. Vomiting
4. Weakness
5. Weight loss

WHAT TO DO TO EASE YOUR LOVED ONE'S PAIN AND DISCOMFORT (BESIDES THE GENERAL GUIDELINES AT THE BEGINNING OF THE CHAPTER)

1. Use compound antiemetic medication for nausea.
2. Use pain medication for pain (usually morphine).

3. Pace activities to preserve energy.

4. Use a stool softener and gentle laxative to help move bowels.

5. Get emotional support due to the quick diagnosis and prognosis.

DEMENTIA/ALZHEIMER'S DISEASE

Dementia is a general term for a decline in mental ability that's severe enough to interfere with functions of daily living. Alzheimer's disease accounts for 60 to 80 percent of dementia cases. Brain lesions called amyloid plaques accumulate, causing a declining ability to cope as brain cells die. It's a neurodegenerative disorder, and people can live an average of seven to fourteen years after the initial diagnosis.

Approximately 4.5 million Americans suffer from this disease, which usually begins after age sixty. It first shows up as loss of memory. Next to be affected are the person's emotions and inhibitions.

Unfortunately, dementia can't be cured and is a tremendous burden on caregivers physically, psychologically, and emotionally. Someone has to be with the patient 24/7 because otherwise they might inadvertently harm themselves or get out of the house and become lost.

Dementia is also especially difficult because many of the symptoms mimic what we see in people at end of life. But with a dementia patient, these might not actually signal end of life. For example, some signs that someone may be entering the transition phase include sleeping most of the time, talking to people who aren't there, and incontinence. However, these can also be symptoms at the *early* stages of dementia.

So how do we know when a dementia patient is nearing the end and qualifies for hospice care? Generally, they won't be allowed a hospice nurse or admission to a hospice facility unless there has been a decrease in food intake that can be measured in weight loss. The weight loss also needs to continue for someone to receive covered hospice services. Dementia is one of the most common disease processes from which people "graduate" (or get kicked off, as many families feel) from hospice services. Unfortunately, it's also a disease that makes families need lots of support.

It's imperative to have support, because no one can care for someone with dementia on their own. I once visited a woman who had little help and was carrying most of the weight of her mother's care alone. She told me that once, she broke down crying at her mother's bedside. Her mother put her hand on her daughter's head and said, "Don't cry, Lisa." Her mother hadn't spoken in years, but she heard the crying and had a brief moment of lucidity, even remembering her beloved daughter's name. It was a moment of grace in the midst of all the pain.

SYMPTOMS OF DEMENTIA/ALZHEIMER'S DISEASE

1. Cognitive changes
2. Memory loss, which means difficulty remembering recent events or conversations. While it's normal to forget appointments or names occasionally, people with dementia may forget them more often and not remember them later. They might remember events from long ago, however.

3. Difficulty with complex tasks and challenges with planning or solving problems, such as following a plan or working with numbers

4. Confusion as to time and place. This often involves losing track of dates, seasons, and the passage of time. They may become confused about where they are or how they got there.

5. Difficulty understanding visual images and spatial relationships. This could manifest as trouble reading, judging distance, and determining color or contrast, potentially causing issues with driving.

6. Trouble following or joining conversations. They might stop in the middle of a conversation and have no idea how to continue, or they may repeat themselves.

7. Struggling with vocabulary, such as having trouble finding the right word or calling things by the wrong name

8. Personality changes, such as becoming confused, suspicious, depressed, fearful, or anxious. They may be easily upset at home, with friends, or when out of their comfort zone. They might become paranoid, thinking you or someone else around them is trying to harm them.

9. Withdrawal from work or social activities and showing less interest in hobbies and sports

10. Changes in mood and behavior. They might experience mood swings, anxiety, irritability, or changes in sleep patterns. They might roam around late in the day and at night, which is called "sundowning."

SPECIFIC SAFETY CONCERNS
FOR SOMEONE WHO HAS DEMENTIA

1. High risk for choking on food
2. High risk for aspiration pneumonia (food going into the lungs)
3. High risk for falls
4. High risk for skin breakdown (pressure ulcers from sitting or lying in one position for too long)

WHAT TO DO TO EASE YOUR LOVED ONE'S PAIN AND DISCOMFORT (BESIDES THE GENERAL GUIDELINES AT THE BEGINNING OF THE CHAPTER)

1. Use pain medication when necessary.
2. Serve them soft meals.
3. Use barrier cream on pressure ulcers.
4. Do everything you can to have a support system of several people to rotate your loved one's care.
5. Use music and song to connect with your loved one, as dementia patients often retain this part of their memory.

STROKE

Stroke is the fourth leading cause of death in America and a leading cause of adult disability. A stroke occurs when a blood clot blocks an artery or a blood vessel, interrupting blood flow to an area of the brain. When this happens, brain cells begin to die, damaging the brain. The abilities that were controlled by the damaged area of the brain are lost, either temporarily or permanently. These abilities might include speech, swallowing, movement, and memory.

SYMPTOMS OF STROKE

1. Facial drooping
2. Aphasia, or inability to speak
3. Hemiparesis, or weakness on one side of the body
4. Confusion, suddenly having trouble understanding conversations
5. Trouble seeing with one or both eyes, which may include blurred or blackened vision
6. Difficulty walking, loss of balance, or coordination
7. Dizziness
8. Severe headache with no known cause, sometimes accompanied by vomiting or lapses in consciousness

SPECIFIC SAFETY CONCERNS FOR SOMEONE WHO HAS HAD A STROKE

1. High risk for choking
2. High risk for aspiration pneumonia (food going into the lungs)
3. High risk for falls
4. High risk for skin breakdown (pressure ulcers from sitting or lying in one position for too long)

WHAT TO DO TO EASE YOUR LOVED ONE'S PAIN AND DISCOMFORT (BESIDES THE GENERAL GUIDELINES AT THE BEGINNING OF THE CHAPTER)

1. Use pain medication when necessary.
2. Serve them soft meals.
3. Apply barrier cream to pressure ulcers.
4. Do whatever possible to have a support system of several people to rotate your loved one's care.

COLON CANCER

Also known as colorectal cancer, colon cancer starts in the colon or rectum, which are parts of the gastrointestinal (GI) tract, or digestive system. The digestive system processes food for energy and rids the body of solid waste. Colon cancer typically begins as small, benign clumps of cells called polyps that form inside. Over time, some of these polyps can become cancerous. Note that symptoms may not appear in the early stages of the disease.

This kind of cancer impacts populations around the globe, marking it as one of the leading causes of cancer-related deaths worldwide.

Your loved one will likely feel embarrassed by the odor and mess that sometimes results from this disease. Do your best to maintain their dignity. The tumor in the colon often grows, which causes extreme pressure and pain, necessitating increased doses of morphine.

SYMPTOMS OF COLON CANCER
1. Changes in bowel habits

2. Persistent abdominal discomfort
3. Rectal bleeding or blood in the stool
4. A feeling that the bowel doesn't empty completely
5. Weakness or fatigue
6. Unexplained weight loss

WHAT TO DO TO EASE YOUR LOVED ONE'S PAIN AND DISCOMFORT (BESIDES THE GENERAL GUIDELINES AT THE BEGINNING OF THE CHAPTER)

1. Work closely with health care providers/hospice to ensure tight pain control. As the tumor grows in the colon, it will become very painful, so with this kind of cancer, monitor pain several times a day, as it can change quickly.
2. Passing dark blood and blood clots is common with colon cancer. Maintain your loved one's dignity by having cleaning supplies on hand.
3. Ask them who they are most comfortable with to do the hands-on care.
4. An odor will accompany the blood, so apply a small amount of Vicks VapoRub under your nose to mask the smell.

BRAIN CANCER

This kind of cancer occurs when abnormal cells form in the brain. The tumors might have started in the brain, or they might have spread from somewhere else, which is called brain metastasis.

Common metastatic cancers are breast cancer and especially lung cancer.

This disease can be particularly heartbreaking. I worked with a lovely man who had brain cancer. The family hired a professional health care aide to help, but unfortunately, the aide experienced physical and verbal abuse from the patient. It was a very difficult situation.

Since people with brain cancer are affected cognitively, the tumors can change their behavior and personality, causing them to say and do things they would never have said or done otherwise. It's important to keep this in mind if your loved one has brain cancer.

Your loved one will likely require a variety of medications due to the different symptoms that present with brain cancer. It can be a very difficult disease to handle, so tight symptom management is vital.

SYMPTOMS OF BRAIN CANCER
1. Headache
2. Nausea
3. Vomiting
4. Difficulty breathing/shortness of breath
5. Anxiety from shortness of breath
6. Rapid respiratory rate as the body tries to get more oxygen
7. Increased pulse rate from the heart trying to get more oxygen into the body
8. Altered state of consciousness
9. Vision impairment
10. Seizures

11. Hemiparesis, or weakness on one side of the body
12. Cognitive impairment
13. Behavioral and personality changes
14. Seizures

WHAT TO DO TO EASE YOUR LOVED ONE'S PAIN AND DISCOMFORT (BESIDES THE GENERAL GUIDELINES AT THE BEGINNING OF THE CHAPTER)

1. Work closely with health care providers/hospice to ensure tight pain control. With this kind of cancer, monitor pain several times a day, as it can change quickly.
2. Have nausea and seizure medication ready, if needed.
3. Use supplemental oxygen for shortness of breath.

ADVANCED BREAST CANCER

This kind of cancer causes the growth of malignant cells in the breast tissue. It's one of the most common cancers affecting women worldwide, although it can also occur in men. Understanding breast cancer, its risk factors, symptoms, and treatment options is essential for early detection and effective management. When caught early, it's often treatable.

Breast cancer has two main categories:

1. Noninvasive (in situ) breast cancer. The cancerous cells remain in a particular location of the breast without spreading to surrounding tissue.

2. Invasive (infiltrating) breast cancer. The cancerous cells break through normal breast tissue barriers and spread to other parts of the body through the bloodstream or lymph nodes. End-stage invasive breast cancer that metastasizes commonly spreads to the brain.

Many times, someone will have breast cancer for years or even decades before it enters the advanced stage and end-of-life experience.

SYMPTOMS OF ADVANCED BREAST CANCER

1. Pain, including severe neck and/or back pain
2. Fatigue
3. Seizures
4. Emotional and mood changes
5. Digestive issues

WHAT TO DO TO EASE YOUR LOVED ONE'S PAIN AND DISCOMFORT (BESIDES THE GENERAL GUIDELINES AT THE BEGINNING OF THE CHAPTER)

1. Use liquid morphine and Ativan for pain management and shortness of breath.
2. Use seizure medication when necessary.
3. Pace activities to preserve energy.
4. Use a stool softener and gentle laxative to help move bowels.

AMYOTROPHIC LATERAL SCLEROSIS (ALS)

ALS, also known as Lou Gehrig's disease, is a progressive neuro-degenerative disease that affects nerve cells in the brain and spinal cord. ALS leads to a gradual decline in muscle control, impacting physical function over time. It doesn't affect cognitive ability, however, so people with this disease are aware of what's happening to them.

I worked with a man who had ALS, and he told me that when the disease got bad enough, he would "take care of it," meaning he would find a way to end his life. Of course, that might not be possible if paralysis sets in. But I assured him that his family would be taught how to administer higher doses of morphine to keep him comfortable in a palliative coma, even when he began to struggle with breathing. I wanted to alleviate his fear and help him feel safe. So I showed him the bottle of liquid morphine that was in his house and explained just how many milligrams were in the bottle. There would be plenty to take care of him. He was comforted by this knowledge, and as a result, he had a gentle and good death.

Recognizing the symptoms early can be crucial for managing the condition.

EARLY SYMPTOMS OF ALS

1. Muscle weakness, often first noticed in one arm, leg, or foot and described as a subtle change, such as difficulty buttoning a shirt, writing, or tripping while walking. Sometimes it begins as a foot drop, which is difficulty lifting the front part of the foot.

2. Muscle twitches (fasciculations), such as small, involuntary muscle contractions visible under the skin

3. Tight and stiff muscles (spasticity) that lead to muscle cramps and discomfort

4. Difficulty speaking or swallowing. Speech may become slurred (dysarthria), and swallowing (dysphagia) can become challenging as the disease progresses.

5. Fatigue, especially in the muscles of the arms and legs

LATER SYMPTOMS AS ALS PROGRESSES

1. Increased muscle weakness, affecting mobility, grip strength, talking, swallowing, and breathing

2. Breathing difficulties due to weakening of the respiratory muscles, leading to the need for a ventilator

3. Difficulty holding the head up, resulting from weakness in the neck muscles

4. High risk for skin breakdown (pressure ulcers)

5. High risk for aspiration pneumonia (food going into the lungs)

WHAT TO DO TO EASE YOUR LOVED ONE'S PAIN AND DISCOMFORT (BESIDES THE GENERAL GUIDELINES AT THE BEGINNING OF THE CHAPTER)

1. Use liquid morphine and Ativan for pain management and shortness of breath.

2. Try nonpharmacological methods, such as massage or warm baths.

3. Use supplemental oxygen or other breathing aids to ease breathing difficulties.

4. Physical therapists can suggest devices or techniques to maintain mobility and comfort as long as possible, such as adjustable beds, wheelchairs, and cushions.

5. As swallowing becomes more challenging, offer small meals of soft foods and thickened liquids to avoid choking.

6. Speech therapists can provide strategies and tools to facilitate communication, even as verbal abilities decline.

7. Use technology and speech-generating devices that enable communication, allowing your loved one to express their needs, thoughts, and feelings. You can also use a letter board, or ask your loved one to blink their eyes for yes.

Taking care of someone at end of life is a very meaningful experience, but it can also take a tremendous toll on the caregiver. With that in mind, let's talk next about how you, as a caregiver, can guard against burnout.

How Caregivers Can Avoid Burnout

Caring for myself is not self-indulgence, it is self-preservation.

—Audre Lorde

knew a wonderful woman who used social media to share the journey of her father's end of life in real time. It was obvious their relationship was special. Being his main caregiver, she talked online about the types of care she was providing and the sudden, scary, and poignant moments along the way. Then she shared that her father had taken his last breath surrounded by family who loved him dearly.

Suddenly, after that announcement, she went silent. There were no posts for weeks. Finally, she posted again that as her father's body was being driven away from the funeral home, she fainted and ended up in the hospital. After further assessment, they discovered that she hadn't eaten or even consumed much water in many days. She was completely depleted and dehydrated.

I wish I could say this was an anomaly, but it happens to caregivers all the time. It even has a name now: caregiver syndrome. And it's a silent epidemic because so many countries have inadequate elder care and end-of-life care, but it can happen even in countries that have excellent available care.

It's common at the end of life for a family member to suddenly be thrown into full responsibility for the care of their dying loved one. Most of the time, they don't know the first thing about how to do that or how to navigate their country's health care system to get the support they need. Hospice services help tremendously, but in most places in the world, the family is still responsible for the majority of hands-on care. Often, caregivers are adult children of elderly parents, who fall into what we call the "sandwich generation." This means they may also have young children at home who need them at the same time that their parents reach end of life. The degree of obligation and stress that falls on their shoulders can feel like the size of the *Titanic*.

I have watched caregivers suffer from physical ailments, as well as depression, despair, anxiety, guilt, anger, resentment, and, of course, grief. All of these feelings are normal, but they can become debilitating if we aren't careful.

And you'd think a hospice nurse would be immune to such a thing, wouldn't you? We would know better than to allow burnout to happen. But no, this same thing even happened to me during my career.

I was caring for a little boy at the end of his life. The case was so difficult that it pushed all of the medical staff to their limits. In spite of everything, he did have a good death, but whenever we lose someone so young, it's particularly heartbreaking.

Right after his death, I got very ill, and my face became paralyzed. I went to a neurologist, and they said the MRI showed that my cranial nervous system was so inflamed that it lit up like Christmas lights. In addition to the facial paralysis, I had horrible headaches that left me in so much pain that I often cried uncontrollably. The neurologist actually said, "Go home and get your affairs in order." But thankfully, he was wrong about my prognosis. My recovery was slow, but I did recover.

In retrospect, I know this happened because of how much I pushed myself while caring for that little boy. I was so intent on doing everything I could for him and for his family that I didn't take care of even my basic needs. I neglected myself to the point that I put my own health in dire jeopardy.

Case in point: I once asked a group of surviving spouses about their biggest regrets, and their top two were (1) "not caring for myself better when my loved one was ill" and (2) "not asking for help from family, friends, and others."

Those are my regrets, too. In fact, there were nurses available to me, and I could have asked them for more assistance. But I didn't. I wasn't comfortable asking them, and maybe I didn't want to admit I needed help. Well, that experience taught me a big lesson that I never had to learn again, and my hope is that I can spare you the same. Caregiver burnout is real and serious. You can truly harm yourself if you don't pay attention to what you need. It's that important.

SELF-CARE IS *NOT* SELFISH!

We are taught in our society that we're supposed to sacrifice ourselves for others. We're supposed to give and give and give until we're empty, run-down, and ill. How does this make sense? We expect ourselves to be superhuman, but no matter how "super" any of us may be, none of us is Wonder Woman or Superman. And self-care isn't selfish or self-indulgent.

If you're caring for someone else who needs you, that's when it's *most* important to also take care of yourself. This means making time for your own needs, eating properly, getting exercise, ensuring you get enough sleep, and taking care of yourself mentally and emotionally. You will need time to yourself and moments to recharge. Even a couple of hours to nap or have lunch with a friend can help boost your morale.

If you don't do this, you will suffer, and your loved ones might end up suffering as well because of it. You won't be able to make sound decisions, and you'll be much more likely to lose your temper with them or with the other people involved, causing long-term damage to your relationships.

No one benefits when we try to be martyrs. When we pour from a dry pitcher, all we have to offer anyone else is sand. When we instead fill our own pitcher first until it overflows, we have a surplus to give to others. So when you take care of yourself, you are—by extension—caring for your loved ones. Self-care allows you to be the healthiest, most vibrant, and most present caregiver possible.

You will also need to set boundaries with others who might expect more from you than you can give. I know someone who struggled with this while she was her mother's legal guardian at the end of her mother's life. Other loved ones cried on her shoulder constantly, expecting her to help them through their grief and answer all of their questions about her mother's condition. She had nobody to help her through her own grief, and she felt she had to listen to everyone else's pain even though she was exhausted and emotionally spent. She didn't have the bandwidth to always be there for everyone else, and she wasn't honest with herself about that. Eventually, she snapped and screamed at her aunt, which caused tension between them.

While it isn't easy to strike a balance between self-care and caring for someone who needs us a great deal, it's necessary to strive for that balance as much as we can. It's only then that we can make sure we will be available for others. But beyond that, we are each worthy of the same care and love that we provide to someone else. Of course, this doesn't mean that we should put more pressure on ourselves to be "perfect" at self-care. *Just do your best to be gentle with yourself every day.*

ASKING FOR HELP IS YOUR *GREATEST* STRENGTH

I always say that end-of-life care should not and cannot be done by one person. So why are we so stubborn about asking for help? We have been told it's weak to need help. We've been taught it's selfish (there's that word again), and we're afraid we'll be turned down and feel hurt. We think no one else will care as much or do it as well as we can. So we trudge through and try to make it on our own. But as I learned the hard way, it's such a foolish decision. Most people genuinely want to help. Think about it: You like to help, and it makes you feel good when you can. Don't others deserve that feeling as well?

It actually takes *strength* to ask for help. Yes, we have to risk rejection, and we have to admit to ourselves and others that we are actually *not* Wonder Woman or Superman. It means we have to show our vulnerability, and that's a strength as well. It takes courage to let go of the pretense that we're invincible or perfect. Of course, nobody is invincible or perfect, and the smartest people rely on others for help.

If you ask someone for assistance and they turn you down, move on. Resist the urge to label them as "selfish," just as you wouldn't want someone to give you that label. We all have different abilities and capacities, and no matter how close we are to someone, we can't know about everything they're dealing with in their life. If they can't offer help, they aren't the best person for the job. You want someone who has the capacity and willingness to do things for you with a sense of joy and caring.

You may also feel that you shouldn't have to ask for help. "People should be offering their help to me," you might think. But the truth is that people don't know what you need unless you tell them, and you need to be specific about what they can provide you. In my case with my young hospice patient, I thought it was obvious how much I needed help, but when I asked the nurse who was supposed to back me up why she never helped, she said, "You never asked." Boom! There you have it.

So if you could use someone to bring you dinner a couple of nights a week, ask them! I'll bet there are people in your life who would be more than happy to do that for you or to go grocery shopping for you once a week. Think of the ways someone else could take a task off your plate and free up some time for you to decompress, take a hot bath, or spend a few minutes sitting quietly in the park listening to the birds. Even people who are far away can help by lending an ear on the phone, helping out with paperwork, or contributing financially, if needed and possible.

I realize some of you may be reading this and thinking, "But I really don't have anyone to ask." I understand. It may be that you feel truly on your own in your caregiving tasks, but I ask you to think again about where you might be able to get help.

I know someone who felt she had few people to ask for help, and that made it difficult for her. "Others I knew just didn't have the capacity to help me with paperwork, research, or phone calls, but I *could* lean on them for emotional support. I could ask them to simply let me vent, and that made a big difference," she told me. One of the most important things you can have as a caregiver is someone who will just listen without judgment or agenda.

If you don't have people in your life who can listen when you need an ear, search for groups online of other caregivers who understand what you're going through. Sometimes, just spending ten to fifteen minutes chatting with someone online who understands it all can take a huge amount of pressure off of you. It allows you to debrief and honor your emotions. It's like an energetic cleanse, which we all need on a regular basis (even when we aren't in a caregiving situation). So never underestimate the impact of an understanding ear. The power of presence is the best medicine we have to give to one another. In the Resources section at the end of this book, you will find information for joining the Doulagivers Free Family Caregiver Community on Facebook. Many people also use the website CaringBridge.com, which allows them to regularly share with others (privately) about the state of their loved one's condition, and they can also set up a "meal train" or ask friends and family members to help out with certain chores.

When I was involved as a hospice nurse, I often worked with social workers to find local resources to help caregivers. If there's a social worker involved in your situation, they may be an excellent resource to get you help. Some hospice programs also provide short-term assistance to give caregivers a respite from the day-to-day work of caring for someone. There may be elder care or end-of-life Doulagivers in your area who could help as well.

This also helps patients who might feel guilty about being so helpless and requiring so much of the caregiver. Many patients have expressed this guilt to me, so respite care can be a relief for them as well.

Whatever you do, I implore you to begin to think of asking for help as a strength, not a weakness. Grant yourself that grace, and allow others to give you help and love. It might just change your life. With that in mind, let me introduce the Support System Scheduler to make accepting help a practical reality.

CREATE YOUR SUPPORT SYSTEM SCHEDULE

The purpose of the Support System Scheduler is to give you a way to have family, friends, or hired help "fill in" blocks of support time during each week. Let people know that you are happy to have their help for a block of two to four hours or, if possible, an entire shift of eight, twelve, or twenty-four hours. This help, in whatever capacity you have it, will allow you time to restore and rejuvenate your energy and nervous system.

First, make a list of your helpers:

NAME OF CAREGIVER	RELATIONSHIP	PHONE NUMBER	EMAIL ADDRESS
1.			
2.			
3.			
4.			
5.			

Then, see the next page for the Support System Scheduler, and create your schedule:

THE SUPPORT SYSTEM SCHEDULER

Date: _____

Week from: _____   To: _____

	Sunday	Monday	Tuesday	Wednesday	Thursday	Friday	Saturday
1am							
2am							
3am							
4am							
5am							
6am							
7am							
8am							
9am							
10am							
11am							
12pm							
1pm							
2pm							
3pm							
4pm							
5pm							
6pm							
7pm							
8pm							
9pm							
10pm							
11pm							
12am							

For printable versions of the caregiver/helper list and Support System Scheduler, visit Doulagivers.com/comfort-kit and Doulagivers .com/support-system-scheduler/, respectively.

WHO IS *YOUR* CAREGIVER?

Now that I've hopefully convinced you to ask for help, I will ask you to take it a step further. I urge you to do everything you can to find someone who can be *your* caregiver as you are providing care to your loved one. This is your go-to person who can do things for you physically and be there for you emotionally. Of course, if you have lots of needs, it's even better if you have two or three caregivers for yourself!

Again, if you've been taught that requesting help is selfish, work on erasing that lesson from your mind. The better you're able to take care of yourself, the better you'll be able to take care of your loved one at end of life. Find those special people who are willing and have the bandwidth to be there for you. There may come a time when they're in your shoes, and you can return the favor to them.

HOW ARE YOU DOING *REALLY*?

Answer the following questions, and be honest:

1. How are you doing *really*?
2. Are you tired?
3. Are you sleeping okay?

4. Are you eating enough, and is the food you're eating nutritious?
5. Do you feel useful and needed?
6. Are you getting enough support from other family members?
7. Are you getting out of the house enough and having enough time for yourself?
8. Do you feel trapped by your situation?
9. Do you feel overwhelmed?
10. Do you have frequent crying spells?
11. Do you feel edgy and irritable?
12. Do you struggle to concentrate and make decisions?
13. Do you feel lonely or alone?
14. Do you tend to forget to take your own medications?
15. Do you have back pain, headaches, or digestive problems?
16. Do you spend time outside each day?
17. Do you spend any time during the week doing something you enjoy?

Whenever a caregiver answers too many of these questions in a way that shows their stress level is too high, I encourage them to get help and see their own doctor for a checkup.

I strongly recommend daily check-ins, asking yourself how you're doing every morning and evening, with special notice given to eating enough, drinking enough water, sleeping enough, getting support, finding opportunities to vent with someone else, and getting enough time for yourself. If you don't check in with yourself regularly, you can fall into self-neglect far too easily.

YOUR SELF-CARE CHECKLIST

Below is a list of things you can try to help you recharge. Whenever you feel overwhelmed and on the verge of burning out, refer to this chapter and this list.

1. **Ask for help.** I can't say this too many times. You cannot and should not do this alone. Don't be afraid to ask for what you need from others. People often want to help.

2. **Spend time in nature.** Even a five-minute walk outside each day can help. Notice the sunlight, the plants, and the birdsong.

3. **Practice breathing techniques.** Sitting quietly and either meditating or just taking a few deep breaths can be extremely beneficial to you. When you start to feel anxious or overwhelmed, sit down and consciously slow down your breathing. It will help more than you think!

4. **Fill a large water bottle in the morning and make sure you finish it during the day.** Try to drink at least two liters of fresh water per day.

5. **Keep convenient and quality foods around the house at all times.** Drinks like Boost and Ensure (milk chocolate is my favorite) are good sources of protein, vitamins, minerals, and energy when you have little time. Consider making or buying a nutritious casserole or big pot of soup that you can eat for the week—or ask a friend to make one for you!

6. **Turn off your phone and unplug whenever you can.** Try to find at least two short periods of time to do this daily.

7. **Move your body.** Even that five- to fifteen-minute walk in nature can do wonders, but I also suggest some light stretching for ten minutes each day. If you struggle to sleep, this can help if you do it at night. Just don't do it vigorously; keep your stretches relaxed. For each stretch, count to at least thirty.

8. **Listen to your favorite music.** Soft music might help you relax, but loud music can also be cathartic. Maybe what you need is a dance break or a sing-along!

9. **Blow some bubbles.** Playfulness can help us laugh and decompress more than anything. This is a great activity to do with a child.

10. **Make an art project on your own.** If painting, sculpting, crafting, or something else gives you solace, make time for it.

11. **Watch some comedy.** Again, laughter is wonderful medicine and can take us out of our own circumstances.

12. **Go to a movie.** Immersing yourself in another world can give you a respite from your own situation.

13. **Spend time with animals.** If you have pets, spend time with them for comfort, play, and laughter. If you don't have pets, ask to spend time with someone else's pets, or visit a local farm or petting zoo.

14. **Get a baby monitor.** If you keep a monitor in your loved one's room, it can give you peace of mind when you need to spend time alone elsewhere in the house.

In the next chapter, we will review the options for funerals and wakes.

6

The Rebirth of Death

Anyone who can operate a washcloth can do
a home funeral for a loved one.
—Lee Webster, former president of the National
Home Funeral Alliance

As I picked up the phone, the soft, familiar voice on the other end said, "I need you to come over to my apartment this week. Can you come Tuesday afternoon at three?" It was my dear friend Shatzi Weisberger. Ninety years old at the time and less than five feet tall, Shatzi was still a force to be reckoned with. She was a former registered nurse, a fearless death educator, and my cohost of our Death Café in New York City for three years. (A Death Café is a scheduled nonprofit get-together for the purpose of talking about death over food and drink, usually tea and cake. The idea originated with the Swiss sociologist and anthropologist Bernard Crettaz, who organized the first *café mortel* in 2004.) I could hear some urgency in her request, but I didn't ask why. I only wondered to myself, "What is this about?"

When Shatzi opened the door that Tuesday and hugged me, she immediately started pointing out everything in her apartment that was to be given away and to whom. She had placed stickers every-where with the names of the proper recipients. "I thought of these two things for you," she said as she indicated a beautiful hall mirror and a painting of a young girl in a countryside meadow at sunset. "Just tell me what you want," she said.

As we walked by a chest in the living room, she pointed out the clothes that were carefully folded on the end of the wooden bench. "This is the outfit I'm going to be buried in," she said with pride. It was a coral-pink floral shirt and white pants. Then she told me the names of the friends who would care for her in her final days. Her immediate after-death plan included rituals of prayer and celebra-tion, the food that would be brought in for those joining her home wake, and the music that would be played. She had considered every detail.

She had also meticulously planned and prepaid for a serene nat-ural burial at a cemetery just ninety minutes north of New York City. Every wish was carefully documented by the compassionate funeral director. The only uncertainty that remained was when this poignant farewell would occur, since Shatzi was still in impeccable health.

As she outlined her plans, there was not only a feeling of empow-erment coming from my friend, but one of complete confidence as well. I had never experienced anything like it before. Shatzi was always an inspiration for me in life, and it was clear she would be an inspiration for me in death as well.

Since we can't change the fact that death will be a part of all our lives, is the answer to follow Shatzi's example and change our per-spective of death? Change it to an empowered celebration of a life well lived with many more choices than the usual ones about how to celebrate it? Could the day we die be looked at as another birth? I know many people believe this. What if it were considered our second birthday?

More traditional ways of dealing with death are having a rebirth around the world, and as a result, people are experiencing empowerment and emotional healing through making their own choices for ritual and ceremony. They are going back to their roots with the readoption of home wakes and funerals. Centuries ago, this was the common way to handle death. For millennia, people from many cultures would die at home and remain there for the viewing and ceremony to honor their life, regardless of the climate, type of illness, age of the deceased, or traumatic circumstance surrounding the death. The professionalization and commodification of the funeral industry only became popular at the beginning of the twentieth century and spread throughout a substantial portion of the world. Therefore, many people today believe that they have no choice but to hire funeral professionals and that taking care of their own deceased is no longer an option. This is not at all the case.

In this chapter, you'll learn about the various options outside of a "standard" funeral.

THE ANCIENT BENEFITS AND TRANSFORMATIONAL POWER OF THE THREE-DAY HOME WAKE

Brandon was a sixteen-year-old who was the most popular boy in his high school. He was known for being smart, talented, and universally kind to everyone, whether they were popular kids like him or the kids who usually felt invisible except for the care and attention they received from Brandon. Then, suddenly, he suffered a cerebral hemorrhage that took his life in a matter of minutes. It seemed as though the entire population of his school showed up for his short funeral, which was the tradition in his community. But the chapel couldn't handle the numbers, and his fellow students spilled outside the doors. Everyone sobbed audibly, and it was a beautiful ceremony. But the short duration left everyone to go home and deal with their pain on their own.

Then there's Jared—a handsome, beloved seventeen-year-old with an enviable head of curly brown hair and huge brown eyes. He was on the threshold of life when he had a motorcycle accident and died suddenly. Of course, his family and friends were just as devastated as Brandon's, but their decision to bring Jared's body home from the hospital for a home wake that lasted three days made all the difference. His story was told in a documentary film by Heidi Boucher and Ruby Sketchley called *In the Parlor: The Final Goodbye.*

The extraordinary thing about the three-day event was that mourners began the experience dissolved in shattering, inconsolable grief, just as those who attended Brandon's funeral had. But by the third day, something magical happened. Their grief began to transform until they were singing, smiling, and rejoicing about this young man they loved so much. Jared's mother described the feeling of love in their home as "euphoric." Experiences like this can turn death on its head, truly making it a celebration of the person's life.

Most people suffer from traumatic grief even when someone in their nineties dies after a long terminal illness, so how is it possible for grief to transform into jubilation in just three days' time after the sudden death of a seventeen-year-old?

The tradition of holding a wake for three days after someone's death is deeply rooted in a variety of cultures and religions worldwide. In Irish custom, the wake is one of the oldest death rituals, with its origins likely traced back to ancient Jewish practices of leaving the burial chamber unsealed for three days. The Greek Orthodox tradition also includes a three-day wake called the Panikhida, during which family and friends recite the Book of Psalms. For Thai Buddhists, a short funeral is inconceivable. They spend three days or more, ending with cremation on the last night.

This period allows relatives to pay their respects, share memories, and often engage in traditional songs and games to honor the deceased.

Some believe three days give the soul or spirit of the deceased time to fully let go of their physical body, while others report that they can feel the presence of the person who died during the three-day funeral.[1] In these kinds of ceremonies, the person's spirit often feels omnipresent, almost like they are there, embracing everyone in attendance in their love and energy.

Regardless of someone's beliefs, these ancient traditions underscore the importance of community and collective grieving in the face of death. They can mean the difference between staying stuck in despair or moving on with fond, joyful memories. They provide a structured outlet for expressing grief and honoring the continuity of life that's difficult to replicate in a one-hour or two-hour ceremony.

While, of course, not everyone is capable of having a ceremony for three days, knowing about these customs can help us create more compassionate, empathetic, and inclusive end-of-life experiences, allowing us to better support everyone who is navigating through the loss. Even if it isn't possible to spend several days together, it's helpful to spend as much time together as possible to tell stories about the deceased person, such as in the Jewish tradition of sitting shiva. While traditional shiva originally lasted for seven days, modern shiva may look more like visiting hours for a few hours on a select day or days, depending on the observers' preferences and responsibilities. This time, whether days or hours, can give people a healing outlet for their grief, making it easier to move forward.

At wakes, some people include photo boards that chronicle the person's life, home videos, audio recordings, or the deceased's artwork. I know of one case where the family had a life-size standing replica made of their son, who died of AIDS in his twenties. At his memorial service, people took selfies with it, which was so in keeping with his sense of humor. I'm thinking of having a dancing flash mob at mine! There are many opportunities to bring celebration into wakes and funerals, regardless of their length.

THE BENEFITS OF A HOME FUNERAL

People have found that home funerals can afford them many advantages. For one, the grieving can slow down and be truly present to take in the sacred moments of not only grief and remembrance, but spiritual connection with family and friends. When a funeral is held in a formal funeral home, families are often rushed through the ceremony, and they have to follow strict protocols that they don't have to follow at home.

A home funeral also allows us to exercise environmental responsibility by foregoing invasive and toxic procedures like embalming and postmortem makeup that can make the deceased look unnatural. This is especially important, of course, if the body is to be viewed during the ceremony in a casket, box, bed, or on a table. At a home funeral, the body is washed and dressed or covered, and then usually preserved for the three days (or whatever length) using dry ice or Techni-Ice, which is safe and reusable. (Note that the body must be dressed soon after death because it will begin to stiffen within a few hours.)

The home is usually a comforting place rather than a foreign one, which brings healing to the family and community. Plus, there is something empowering about caring for our loved ones ourselves rather than outsourcing the responsibility to someone else. It can perhaps serve as our last expression of love for this person, as well as a family rite of passage that is more meaningful for all involved.

People often choose to have guests decorate the box, casket, or cremation urn in honor of the deceased. This is a wonderful way to allow children to participate in a loving, fun, and transformative way, helping to allay their fear of death.

The cost of a standard funeral averages $7,848 in the United States in 2023, according to a National Funeral Directors Association study.[2] On the other hand, a home funeral costs the price of the dry ice (if used), the additional cost of food for a reception, gasoline when transporting the body, and a rigid container, such as a cardboard box or pine casket, usually totaling less than $200.

In contrast to a home funeral, when someone's body is removed from the hospital by the coroner, it's placed in a plastic bag and wheeled away on a gurney, which can be a chilling last visual image. On numerous occasions, I have assured families that I would see to it their loved one was treated gently when removed from the hospital. Most US states allow families to take the deceased directly home from the hospital, but you must check the laws in your state or country. Some places may require you to use a professional funeral home for some of the tasks needed to care for the dead.

Of course, burial or cremation costs must be added at the going rate at the local cemetery or facility. But as you can see, beyond the potential emotional and spiritual advantages, a home funeral can offer a considerable economic advantage.

LIVING WAKES/LIVING *FUNERALS*

My friend Mary was just in her thirties when she became terminally ill. So she decided to have a "living wake," during which her family and friends spent time with her to celebrate her life and tell her how much she was loved, appreciated, and admired before she died. It was an extraordinary experience. There are scenes of a similar event in a romantic comedy movie called *Love at First Sight,* in which the male protagonist's terminally ill mother decides to have a Shakespearean-themed pre-death memorial service. Her friends and family arrive in period clothing and are all tasked with performing for her, which they do gladly. It's a beautiful part of the film.

My friend Shatzi did this as well when she turned ninety-two. She knew that time was running out and thought, "Why not?" She coined it her "FUNeral." She used it to make the death transition a vibrant party, where death was embraced with joy and curiosity. One hundred souls gathered in her apartment building's community room, indulging in delectable food and drink, while adorning a biodegradable cardboard coffin with messages of love for Shatzi. The air was filled with live music, dancing, and heartfelt conversations about the profundity of death. Clad in white, Shatzi radiated peace and wisdom as she shared her insights on her inevitable journey, showcasing the beauty of embracing mortality. It was the epitome of a good death celebration.

A living wake or living funeral is generally the same type of ceremony as a traditional wake or funeral except it happens before the person has died. It's a chance for a community of friends and family to come together and express the impact their loved one has made on their lives while they are still around to hear it. And it's a chance for someone who might feel out of control to take back some control.

Why shouldn't we be able to hear all the wonderful things people would say about us after we're gone? It's an opportunity to say final goodbyes, offering everyone a chance to leave nothing unsaid and to feel a sense of closure.

In Shatzi's eternally life-affirming spirit, I recommend genuinely having fun with FUNerals. Pick the venue, the food, and the eighties music (or is that just me?), and invite everyone your loved one wants to be there. It can be done on a small budget in a backyard with everyone bringing their signature potluck dishes. It's a wonderful way to ease the pain of dying and commemorate a life well lived.

EULOGIES WRITTEN IN FIRST PERSON

A eulogy is a heartfelt tribute, usually delivered at a funeral or memorial service, to honor and celebrate the life of the person who has died. The clergy or someone close to the deceased generally performs the eulogy, which is an opportunity to share memories, express feelings, and acknowledge the significance of the deceased's life. But there is a new trend where the dying person writes their own eulogy in the first person prior to their death so that it can be read by a loved one at their funeral.

I have never felt more love and healing than when a room full of people, grieving the death of someone they love, get to hear from that person directly in their first-person eulogy. It's one of the most powerful things I have ever experienced, and I have experienced it a lot. It allows everyone to feel that their loved one is still with them.

Below is such a eulogy written in first person:

> The idea of writing your own eulogy is daunting, but I love the idea of having the last word.
>
> All joking aside, what I truly love about this is getting to tell you all how I feel about you after I'm gone, or at least appear to be gone. I firmly believe that I'm still here with you. It's just that you can't see me anymore. I always did want to be invisible, so I guess now is my chance.
>
> First of all, I want you all to know how much you mean to me. Each and every one of you has had a positive impact on my life—even though we may not have gotten along at every moment. And to my wife and kids, you were and are everything to me. There are no words to express what you brought to my life, and I'm so grateful to have had each of you. I was one very lucky guy. You were the sun, the moon, and all the planets and stars. I promise to watch over you forever. And when it's your time to join me, I will welcome you with heavenly kisses and hugs.
>
> I know my illness put you through a lot, but I'm

amazed by how you handled it all with such grace. As you walk through your days without me there physically, just know that I'm still supporting you and loving you no matter what.

Do I wish I could have stayed around to meet my grandchildren? Sure. But I will know them from afar, and I will watch over them, too.

I'm also grateful that I had a chance to say good-bye to everyone while I was still with you physically. That was an enormous blessing. All of you who visited me, I want you to know it meant so much. And if you didn't get a chance to visit me, that's perfectly okay. I can feel your love, and I appreciate it more than you know.

I want to say thank you to everyone for making my last weeks and days so peaceful and truly beautiful in many ways. While it was painful to say good-bye, it was also so profound and spiritual and sacred. I've never experienced anything else like it, and it seems fitting that my last experience in a body would be so expansive, mind-opening, and heart-opening.

As for regrets, I've had a few, as the song lyric said. I regret losing my temper, not reaching out as often as I could have, not telling people I loved them as much as I should have. As most of you know, I could be really stubborn, and I had a temper. Sometimes, I was unyielding, and I could be unforgiving at times, too. I regret wasting time with pride and lack of forgiveness.

If I'm going to offer you any advice, it would be to put your ego aside and just love everything and everyone as much as you can. It would be to enjoy every moment you can to the fullest. In the midst of whatever brings you pain, don't forget to notice all the beauty that exists. There's a lot of it if you just look.

I have also regretted not doing some of the things I always wanted to do. But from my perspective now, as I sit and write this in my last days, what I didn't do no longer matters much. From this vantage point, I really did live a full life, and my bucket list is complete. All of my previous complaints are in the past. I let them go like little balloons in the sky.

Besides, what I did get to do was a lot. I got to have a career that went beyond what I ever thought I'd accomplish. And I got to travel to some beautiful places. I got to express myself through my painting, and I got to appreciate the art that others created.

All of that was wonderful. But nothing compares to the extraordinary family I got to be part of and all the moments I got to spend with the people in my life. That's what I'm carrying with me the most.

When I was young, I dreamed of wealth, greatness, and fame, but now I see that as foolish. It really isn't about the *what*; it's about the *who*. And in that regard, I have been wealthy beyond measure. Seeing the Great Wall of China will never compare to watching my two-year-old perform in the Christmas play.

I hope you'll remember me as someone who tried to be a good person and who loved deeply. Someone who often fell short but came to a place of peace and acknowledgment that love is all that matters.

To my wife, Beth, I knew you were my wife from the minute I saw you at the pep rally the first year of college. And that knowing never changed in all our years of marriage.

To my son, Erik, you have healed parts of me that I never knew were broken. I'm so proud of the man you have become, and I can't wait to have a front row seat from the other side to what you do next.

To my daughter, Jenny, you have become so much more than I could have imagined. Your ability to make me laugh has been unprecedented, and your talent just blows my mind. Always believe in yourself, honey.

To my brother, Griff, I know we haven't always seen eye to eye, but I have always respected you and appreciate the support you've given me. I'll never forget the days spent on the ice together. Live well, you hockey puck.

To my best friend, Phil, thank you for taking over the workload of the business when I got sick and was going through treatment. You allowed me the greatest gift of all: spending these last precious months with my wife and children. You have been an extraordinary partner and ally.

Meanwhile, I ask those of you who are so inclined

to check in with my family periodically to see how they're doing. Maybe in the next few weeks, stop by with a casserole or a pie, or offer to take them somewhere fun.

So I guess my final word has to be thank you to each of you. Picture me standing in front of you, one at a time, telling you how much I appreciate you. Picture me standing in front of you whenever it crosses your mind, reminding you not to give up, to remember you're loved, and to remember to love.

I'll close with a quote from Winnie-the-Pooh: "If there ever comes a day when we can't be together, keep me in your heart. I'll stay there forever."

I love you all.

Of course, your loved one can choose to have more than one eulogy at the funeral or wake. Why not include the words of the deceased, as well as the words of those who love them most?

Exercise: First-Person Eulogy

Using the example in the chapter, ask your loved one to write or dictate a eulogy they would like to be read after their death. Alternatively, they can make an audio recording to be played.

Don't think of this as a sad exercise; think of it as an opportunity for them to speak even when gone. They can have the last word!

Besides the different kinds of funerals discussed in this chapter, there are also several green options today that allow us to keep the environment in mind. That's what we'll talk about in the next chapter, and I will guide you in creating a funeral/wake plan and/or living FUNeral plan.

WRITING AND PUBLISHING AN OBITUARY

Since we've discussed a eulogy, you might be wondering about an obituary. In the past, death notices were usually placed in the newspaper, but since most of our reading is online today, you might submit a death notice or obituary to your local newspaper via email. Note that there is sometimes a charge for this. You might also want to submit it to a college, church, or other organization's publication.

The basics usually include your loved one's full name, age, date of birth and death, cause of death, place of birth, where they lived at the time of their death, the names of survivors, the date and time of the funeral or memorial, and any preferences for expressions of sympathy such as charitable donations.

Today, people often submit to a special obituary website like Legacy.com, which allows people to comment with their condolences and memories of the deceased. This also allows you to include more details about your loved one. Beyond the basics, you might want to add your loved one's work history, their main accomplishments, their main interests, and loving remembrances of them. The answers you receive to the questions from their life review (as discussed in chapter 10) can be helpful for writing a meaningful obituary.

Feel free to write it in an informal style and get input from other members of the family and friends.

7

Keeping Death Green:
How Our Funeral and Burial Choices
Impact the Planet

> Green burial provides a way for bodies to
> rest in nature without disturbance, and with
> reverence.
>
> —Green Burial Council

I sat with Judy on the porch of her picturesque home as she told me about the life she'd lived—what she had learned and what she regretted. While admiring the natural world around us and greeting friendly passersby like the neighborhood postal worker, she also talked about her impending end of life. These talks became a habit for us after I took on the job as her hospice nurse. And every time, it felt like a movie scene.

From my initial visit with Judy, it was crystal clear that this tiny, thin, five-foot-two woman with a long mane of curly silver hair was incredibly grounded and courageous. I could tell she had already come to terms with the fact of her death. She was unfailingly proactive and progressive in making decisions about her end of life.

"They're building a table and pine box casket," she told me.

"I'm going to have a home funeral and then a natural burial. It's all planned." She described this with such strength and peace in her voice that it wasn't like she was talking about death at all.

This is how it should be, I thought. It's so empowering when someone focuses on what they *can* control rather than dwelling on what they *can't*.

Judy was aware of the amazing gifts she had been given throughout her life, and she believed in the importance of showing kindness toward others. She wanted us all to understand our responsibility when choosing options for burial. She felt strongly it should be done as an act of gratitude, with respect not only for ourselves but also for the planet. Natural burial allowed her to express this deep appreciation in the final choice she got to make.

A veteran hospice nurse named Tim placed the call to us with the news. "I just pronounced Judy. Time of death: 6:39 a.m. This was the most beautiful pronouncement I have ever witnessed. Friends and family are gathered in the barn where Judy is laid out in a casket made by a family friend, beautifully adorned with fresh flowers. People are eating and sharing stories of her life. I have never felt anything like this."

Tim had borne witness to much suffering as he pronounced the deaths of patients and broke the news to families he had never met before that moment. His dry and quick-witted sense of humor enabled him to cope with the pain around him while offering solace in those darkest hours.

There is no doubt in my mind that Judy's choice to have a natural burial contributed to her having a good death. She felt wonderful about that decision, and, as an added bonus, her good death touched everyone around her, including a thirty-plus-year hospice nurse.

Unfortunately, most people aren't like Judy. They don't stop to learn about the options that are available to them and consider what they truly want. Yet with a worldwide aging population of more than 761 million—expected to rise to 1.6 billion by 2050[1]—it's more important than ever that everyone chooses their final resting place carefully.

Embalming and standard casket burial have become commonplace without much thought or understanding of their environmental consequences. The toxic chemicals that seep into the soil have a devastating effect on nature's delicate balance, contributing to climate change every time someone is buried conventionally. Many believe that fire cremation is a viable alternative, but this method releases hazardous pollution into the atmosphere. So it's time to rethink our death care practices so that future generations can inherit a healthier planet free from additional human-made destruction due to funeral customs and ceremonies.

In recent years, more and more people are aware of the ecological cost of burial choices. So, like Judy, they're turning toward more traditional methods of honoring the dead. These customs, which include home wakes and natural burials, were a part of our history for centuries before we began to outsource the handling of the dead. We now have choices, and deciding which option is right for us can be one of life's most significant decisions. It can bring us deep peace emotionally, spiritually, and financially when facing the end of life.

The "Dying to Be Green" movement is a growing trend that emphasizes the importance of environmentally sustainable choices. By choosing green options for our body disposition, we can reduce our carbon footprint, conserve natural resources, and support ecosystem health. This movement highlights the need for systemic change in the death care industry as a whole. From reducing waste to advocating for policies that support sustainable death care options, the movement represents a powerful force for positive change at a time when our planet needs it most.

As caregivers, our knowledge of these options allows us to have important conversations with our loved ones about how they want to handle their end of life, while it also allows us to plan ahead for our own good death.

THE HISTORY OF EMBALMING

During the American Civil War, modern embalming emerged as a way to preserve soldiers' bodies so that their loved ones could give them a proper burial at a later date. It isn't at all widespread throughout other parts of the world and is even forbidden in some countries. Yet this custom lives on today in many parts of the US despite its original purpose having long since passed.

Some people mistakenly believe it's legally required after someone dies. It isn't, but there are some exceptions where it may be required or strongly recommended. For example, if a deceased person is being transported across state lines, embalming may be necessary to comply with certain state regulations. Some funeral homes may also have their own policies regarding embalming for open-casket viewings or public visitations. Unfortunately, our lack of death awareness includes a lack of knowledge of our options, rights, and choices. In general, whether due to religious reasons or personal preferences, families have the right to choose whether or not to embalm their loved one and should be informed of *all options* when making end-of-life decisions. And of course, every individual has the right to choose or not choose embalming for themselves ahead of time, and the family should honor that decision even if it does not agree with their own preferences.

CHOICES ARE EMPOWERING

Letting go of our loved ones is never easy, and during times of grief, it can be especially hard to make sound financial decisions while planning a funeral and burial. I recall meeting a woman in Florida who shared how her family had experienced this firsthand when they needed to arrange their father's burial after his death. They were so disoriented by the sudden loss that they ended up splurging on a deluxe casket, extravagant floral arrangements, and even an insurance policy against the casket breaking down. These were all expenses that would have gone against every fiber of the frugal man's being while he was alive. Obviously, not planning ahead can have substantial consequences for us, both emotionally and financially.

Luckily, there are many progressive options for body disposition today. Each method has its own unique set of pros and cons, so it's important to weigh them all carefully before deciding how to proceed. Let's explore what's available.

Nongreen Options
Standard Funeral

A standard funeral typically includes several key components, including embalming of the body, viewing or visitation, a funeral ceremony or service, and burial in a cemetery. (Note that traditional Jewish funerals do not do embalming, and they also allow only a natural-fabric shroud and a casket with no metal parts.)

Pros: Readily available in most places.

Cons: There are several environmental drawbacks to standard embalming and nonbiodegradable caskets:

1. Embalming fluids contain a mixture of chemicals such as formaldehyde, glutaraldehyde, and phenol, which can be harmful to the environment when released into the soil during burial. These chemicals can also pose health risks to funeral home workers who handle them frequently.

2. Nonbiodegradable caskets made of materials like metal or hard wood don't break down naturally in the soil and can take up valuable land space.

3. Traditional burials often involve the use of concrete vaults or liners that are designed to prevent the ground from sinking over time. However, these structures can also prevent natural decomposition and create issues with water runoff.

Cost: The cost of a standard funeral can vary widely depending on a number of factors, such as the location, the funeral home or service provider chosen, and the specific services requested. The average cost of a traditional funeral in the United States is $7,000 to $12,000.

Fire Cremation

Fire cremation is an increasingly popular alternative to traditional burial. The body is placed in a special chamber and exposed to high temperatures that reduce it to ash. The ashes can then be kept in a container or scattered, but there are laws about the scattering of ashes. Check your location for specific laws, but in general in the US, we cannot scatter ashes in a public park without a permit. The federal Clean Water Act requires that the Environmental Protection

Agency be notified before scattering ashes, and if in the ocean, they must be scattered at least three nautical miles out to sea. For lakes and rivers, a permit is usually required from the local government. Ashes can be scattered from the air, but not while still in a container.

Pros: More economical than standard burial, and it grants families flexibility in terms of where ashes may be scattered or stored, while providing convenient transport options during funerals or memorials.

Cons: Even though it's a more environmentally friendly option than traditional burial, it still carries negative environmental impacts:

1. The process of burning the body releases pollutants into the atmosphere such as carbon dioxide, nitrogen oxides, and other toxic gases. A single flame cremation produces an average of 534.6 pounds of carbon dioxide.[2]
2. Fire cremation also emits toxic emissions from mercury or silver dental fillings.
3. These gases and emissions can contribute to air pollution and are thought to be linked to respiratory illnesses such as chronic obstructive pulmonary disease (COPD).

Cost: The average cost of a cremation in the United States is generally less than a traditional funeral. According to the National Funeral Directors Association, the median cost with a memorial service in 2019 was about $5,150, but this figure can vary widely depending on location, type of urn selected, and additional services.

It's worth noting that there are different types of cremation. A "direct" cremation is typically the least expensive option and involves simply transporting the deceased to a crematory for processing without any formal viewing or ceremony beforehand. This can cost as little as $500 to $1,000 in some areas.

Green Options

A green disposition option is a viable way to reduce environmental impact and leave a positive legacy for future generations. Green burial and aquamation, for example, can significantly reduce carbon emissions compared to traditional funeral practices that rely on fossil fuels. Some people may wish to return their remains to nature in order to support ecosystem health and biodiversity. Both human composting and natural burial reserves offer opportunities for families to participate in this process directly.

Cost considerations may also play a role, as green options are less expensive than traditional funerals, making them accessible to people who want to honor their loved one's memory without breaking the bank.

Green/Natural Burial

It's illegal in most places to just bury someone in the woods, and a green/natural burial is much more than that. Typically, the body is wrapped in a biodegradable shroud or placed in a simple wooden casket made from sustainably harvested wood. The grave itself may be left unmarked or marked with natural materials such as stones or plants rather than traditional headstones. These green burials take place in dedicated "green" cemeteries that are specifically designed for this purpose.

Pros: There are several potential benefits of a natural burial:

1. Environmental sustainability: Green/natural burials allow the body to decompose naturally and return to the earth without the use of harmful chemicals or non-biodegradable materials, reducing the environmental impact associated with traditional burial practices.

2. Emotional and spiritual significance: Some people find that a natural burial offers a more meaningful and personal way to say goodbye to their loved one, as it allows for a closer connection with nature and a sense of returning to the earth.

3. Preservation of green spaces: Green cemeteries used for natural burials often serve as protected areas for native flora and fauna, preserving valuable green spaces for future generations.

4. Flexibility and personalization: Natural burials offer greater flexibility in terms of location and ceremony, allowing families to choose a setting that's meaningful to them and personalize the funeral experience in unique ways.

Cons: Not all areas have access to green burial options, so it may not be feasible or practical for everyone. Additionally, some religious beliefs require specific types of burial practices that may not align with natural burial principles.

Cost: These methods are usually less expensive than traditional funerals, as they often involve fewer costly materials and services. The costs vary widely, however, depending on the specific choices made.

Water/Aqua Cremations

Water cremation, also known as aquamation or alkaline hydrolysis, is a new alternative to traditional cremation that involves using water and alkaline chemicals to break down the body. The process is usually carried out in a stainless steel chamber, where the body is placed along with water and potassium hydroxide or sodium hydroxide, which dissolves the tissue over several hours. In the interest of ecology, South African Archbishop Desmond Tutu, who died in 2021, chose this method of disposition for his body upon his death.

Pros: There are several advantages to aquamation:

1. A water cremation uses 90 percent less energy and produces ten times fewer carbon dioxide emissions than a fire cremation. It produces no carbon dioxide or metal emissions.
2. It mimics the natural decomposition of the human body.
3. The liquid byproduct is a nontoxic solution of amino acids, peptides, sugars, and soap, which make a wonderful fertilizer. Families can even take it home to water trees and plants in their personal garden.

Cons: Water cremations aren't legal in every US state yet. As of September 2022, they are legal in the following states:

- Arizona
- California
- Colorado
- Florida
- Georgia
- Idaho

- Illinois
- Kansas
- Maine
- Maryland
- Michigan
- Minnesota
- Missouri
- Nevada
- New Hampshire
- Oregon
- Pennsylvania
- Utah

Cost: Water/aqua cremations cost $2,000 to $3,000.

HUMAN COMPOSTING

Also known as natural organic reduction, human composting is a process that involves converting human remains into soil. It usually means placing the body in a vessel with wood chips, straw, or other organic materials and maintaining it at a specific temperature and moisture level over several weeks to allow for natural decomposition.

During this time, microbes break down the body into its basic components, including carbon, nitrogen, and phosphorus. After the process is complete, what's left is a nutrient-rich soil that can be used for gardening or other purposes.

Pros: Human composting is a more environmentally sustainable alternative to traditional burial or cremation, it involves no chemicals, and it requires less energy than cremation.

Cons: Currently, human composting is legal only in Colorado, Oregon, and Washington State in the US, as well as in the country of Sweden. However, interest in this method is growing, so more states and countries may consider legalizing it in the future.

Cost: Human composting costs $5,000 to $7,000.

BODY DONATION

Also known as whole body donation, this method involves donating the body after death to medical schools, research facilities, or other organizations for medical research and education, such as anatomical study, surgical training, or the development of new medical procedures. Advance arrangements with a specific organization or institution are required. The organization then arranges to transport the body to their facility. As a thank you, many medical schools will hold a "memorial service of gratitude" for families and loved ones of the deceased. After the research has been completed, the medical facility will cremate the remains and return the ashes to the family.

Pros: Some people feel that their death is more meaningful in this case since it will provide a valuable contribution to medicine.

Cons: There are a few considerations with this method:

1. Not all bodies are accepted for donation. Factors such as age, cause of death, and medical conditions may disqualify someone from becoming a donor.
2. It's important to discuss this decision with family members so that they understand and support it.
3. Make sure to find a reputable place for donation. Not all places are equal and may falsely advertise. If you aren't sure, ask doctors and hospitals for advice. In the US, you can search for reputable programs at https://anatbd.acb.med.ufl.edu.

Cost: Free. Once accepted, there is no cost for the donation process, cremation, or return of final remains.

Green Options Often Facilitate a Good Death

In a previous chapter, I told you about the beloved seventeen-year-old, Jared, who was taken from his family, friends, and community after a tragic motorcycle accident. This handsome, six-foot-tall young man with big brown eyes and thick, curly hair was one of those people who left everyone he met feeling seen, heard, and loved—a gift not many of us possess.

Jared's family chose a natural burial for him. Friends and relatives gathered around his body at the home wake, singing songs of love and remembrance, celebrating his life rather than mourning his death. Despite their sorrow over losing such an amazing young man, there was also joy in knowing how much he had been loved by so many people. He was placed in a simple pine coffin, and his family and classmates decorated it with meaningful remembrances of him.

When it came time for the funeral procession, everyone walked together in solemn silence until they reached the nature preserve where Jared would be laid to rest among the trees and birds he had loved since childhood. It felt like a fitting tribute for him to be surrounded by nature's beauty that would never truly die or fade away.

Once everyone arrived at his final resting place, they smiled through their tears as they shared stories about all the wonderful things that made Jared special. His classmates sang joyous songs, and a feeling of peaceful bliss lasted throughout the entire ceremony. Despite having lost someone so dear to them too soon, each person left with a newfound sense of hope.

Green burial options have been proven to have benefits for patients and families emotionally and economically, and they certainly have environmental benefits. We no longer need to settle for traditional burial practices that harm the natural world. These options allow us to come together to create a more sustainable future where both life and death can be celebrated in harmony with nature.

Now, let's begin our Peace of Mind Planner...

PART 2

THE PEACE OF MIND
PLANNER

CHAPTERS 8 TO 12 ARE SIMILAR to a workbook and will function as a practical, holistic A-to-Z planning guide as you initiate important conversations with your loved one and ask them questions about their preferences. The questions will provide you with a thorough plan for your loved one's end-of-life wishes. It includes five categories—physical, mental, emotional, financial, and spiritual—and addresses the majority of concerns that people have expressed to me over my more than twenty years in this field.

The worksheets provided incorporate what you have learned in chapters 1 to 7 about available options, as well as other choices, such as the preferred environment during the final months and days of life. My goal is to leave you with no questions unanswered so that you know exactly what to do when the time comes.

You might think it's too soon to have these conversations or would rather put them off until later, but I encourage you to start now. All too often, I have watched people scramble to figure out what their family member would want, all at the same time that they're frightened, grieving, and scattered. This planner alleviates all of that stress, allowing you to be fully present with the dying person in those last precious moments. It truly does provide peace of mind.

8

A Physical Good Death

Preparing for death is one of the most
empowering things you can do. Thinking
about death clarifies your life.

—Candy Chang

always say that no two end-of-life experiences are the same.
I knew two men, named Rick and Leo, who were both eighty
years old and diagnosed with lung cancer within a month of one
another. But their stories couldn't be more different.

Rick was a well-educated man who had a successful clothing
business and lived in Boston, Massachusetts, with his wife and
two sons. He had a great life with frequent family gatherings, lots
of friends, social events, and vacations. But like many people, he
treated end-of-life planning as though it's optional, never thinking
about it or discussing it with his family.

When he started to experience a persistent cough that lasted for
weeks, he finally went to a doctor. The tests showed that Rick had
stage 4 lung cancer. He and his entire family went into a state of
shock.

Living in Boston, he had access to some of the best medical care available in the US. His oncologist immediately told him, "You need to start chemotherapy right away. Your first treatment will be on Tuesday at 9:00 a.m."

The family consensus was "We need to fight this with everything we've got!" And a whirlwind ensued, with no one pausing to ask the doctors about the odds of success with chemotherapy or the effects of the treatment. The truth was that this was a "fight" with a predetermined winner, and that winner was not Rick.

It also didn't dawn on anyone swept up in the whirlwind to ask Rick what he wanted or to consider any alternatives to what the doctors mandated.

Then there was Leo. Also eighty years old and diagnosed with stage 4 lung cancer, he said to himself, "I've had a good life. I'm just going to go home and live out as many days as I have left in the best way possible."

You see, Leo had given this some thought beforehand. The only son of Tom and Betty, he had been gifted with taking care of his parents, both of whom lived into their nineties but with serious chronic illnesses. He understood the limitations that sometimes come with treatments, and he had accepted the inevitability of end of life.

As a result, he chose exactly where he wanted to be, what activities were important for him to do, who he wanted to care for him, and the final conversations he wanted to have with loved ones. He planned everything from the music that would be played to what would happen to his body after his death and what dishes would be served at his wake.

People told me that toward the end, Leo was busy gardening, visiting with family and friends, and making jokes up until his last week of life.

I saw Rick at several family gatherings during that last year. He was pale, quiet, and weak. Frankly, he looked miserable, scared, and alone. His health took a quick downward turn, and he ended up in hospice care for less than five days. No choices were made. No wishes were honored. And there were no final conversations. His family had remained in the shock phase for a year because no decisions were made that would have allowed them to move into the stabilization phase. Therefore, their traumatic grief was cemented as their final experience with Rick. It was a tremendously sad situation for me to witness and an even more painful one for Rick and everyone who loved him to live through.

We know that with life expectancy now almost double what it was a hundred years ago, the chances that most of us will experience a life-limiting illness are high...and that's okay. What is *not* okay is making uninformed decisions that have dire consequences when we're in the throes of panic, shock, and fear.

The best way I know to diminish those feelings is to make plans *before* a serious diagnosis arrives. Otherwise, we not only leave too much to chance, but we leave our loved ones scrambling at the worst imaginable time to figure out what to do and how to do it. That isn't the kind of legacy any of us wants to leave behind.

While it may feel uncomfortable to think about the possibility of end of life beforehand, consider the relief that will come from knowing that everything has been well planned. Think of the peace everyone will feel not having to guess the wishes of the person when they do reach end of life. Everyone will know exactly what to do, without the stress of trying to figure it out while grieving the inevitable.

Plus, death should be everything the patient wants it to be, and what one person prefers is often the opposite of what someone else wants. We can't know what anyone would like unless we ask them. And no matter how well we think we know someone, I have seen many people be surprised by the answers they received from their loved one. Everyone should get a physical good death.

What specifically is a "physical good death"? It involves four distinct aspects:

1. All physical needs for care at end of life
2. All physical needs at the time of death
3. All physical needs immediately after death
4. All physical needs for disposition of the person's body

This chapter is all about creating a plan for the physical aspects of end of life. I will provide a list of questions in different categories for your loved one to answer to ensure that they have the physical good death they deserve.

QUESTIONS TO ASK THE DOCTOR WHEN THE PATIENT RECEIVES A SERIOUS DIAGNOSIS

It's very difficult for the average person to fully understand medical terminology. Plus, when we first hear a serious diagnosis, the shock can make it hard to take in even the simplest of information. So it's important to ask the proper questions, and I usually recommend that people get a second and even a third opinion before jumping into a treatment plan. It's important to make an informed decision because a hasty or fear-based one can lead your loved one down a path they may not be able to change down the road.

Below are the questions I advise you to ask your loved one's doctor or suggest they ask after receiving a serious diagnosis:

1. How serious/advanced is this? What stage is the disease?
2. What treatments do you suggest?
3. What would my/their overall quality of life look like during the treatment? Would I/they feel sick or weak most of the time?
4. What would happen if I/they chose to do nothing?
5. If chemotherapy is advised, ask the following:

   - With the type of cancer and staging I/they have, are there clinical studies that show how well the chemotherapy worked?
   - How much longer would I/they be likely to live if I/they chose chemotherapy?
   - How long would the treatment be?
   - During the treatment, what side effects would I/they probably experience?
   - How likely am I/they to be hospitalized for chemotherapy complications?
   - Will I/they be unable to do the things I/they enjoy?
   - Would you add any adjunct therapies to chemotherapy, such as Reiki, nutrition plans, vitamins, and/or mineral supplements?
   - Are there alternatives to chemotherapy, and if so, what are they?

Once someone has the answers to these questions, they can make an informed decision about whether chemotherapy or other difficult treatments make sense for them. If the chances of survival are slim even with the treatment, many people, like Leo, opt not to go through it so that they can enjoy the remainder of their life.

CHOICES ABOUT QUALITY OF LIFE

Quality of life is the benchmark for all decisions to be made, but it's subjective. Each person must decide what quality of life means for them. Once they have determined the answer to that question, every other decision should be made from that reference point.

To determine what quality of life means to your loved one, they should make a list—perhaps with your help—of what makes their days worth living. Perhaps it's playing with their pets, watching sports or movies, listening to music, visiting or conversing with certain people, enjoying their favorite foods, or participating in their hobbies or other beloved activities.

There may come a time when your loved one is no longer able to enjoy the things they love, and it's best to have a plan for when that time arrives. Sustaining life through artificial means, surgeries, or procedures that just prolong their existence without quality of life may not align with their desires. Doing so can also sometimes prolong pain and suffering. Being kept alive is different from truly living, and every person needs to set specifications for what they want.

With that in mind, have your loved one answer the following questions, and write down the answers so that you have a record of them. If your loved one can't write their own responses, and you worry that someone else might question the answers, consider recording your loved one vocalizing their answers as you also write them down.

1. What does quality of life mean to you? What activities and people make your days worth living?

_____

_____

_____

2. When quality of life is no longer possible for you, as you have stated above, do you wish your life to be extended through artificial means of feeding, breathing, or other medical interventions? Or would you prefer that these measures *not* be taken to prolong your life?

_____

_____

_____

3. Under what circumstances would you *not* want your life extended? Check all that apply:

- □ I can no longer recognize my loved ones.
- □ I can no longer feed myself.
- □ I am no longer mobile.
- □ I can no longer care for myself with activities of daily living, such as bathing, dressing, eating, and using the toilet.
- □ [Add anything else you wish.]

Based on these choices, this is the time to create a Living Will, POLST, or MOLST, as we discussed in chapter 2.

CHOICES FOR HEALTH CARE PROXY

It's vital that your loved one chooses the *right* person to speak for them if they can't speak for themselves. Everyone needs an advocate at end of life in case they can no longer be their own advocate. The chosen person needs to be a strong, solid support who is willing to abide by the patient's choices without finding it too emotionally trying. As discussed earlier, this person doesn't have to be a family member but must be at least eighteen years old. Ideally, they will reside nearby to easily communicate with doctors and hospital personnel.

A secondary health care proxy must also be chosen in case the first person is unable to serve in that capacity.

Ask your loved one to make these choices carefully, and assist them in creating the health care proxy form.

CHOICES ABOUT END-OF-LIFE CARE

There are so many things that most people don't think about until the moment they become an issue. For example, there usually comes a time when the person near death can no longer bathe themselves or change their clothes. I was serving as a hospice nurse for a woman named Emma who was getting close to that point. We thought she had planned everything out, but the one thing we forgot was specifically designating who would take care of those intimate tasks. I'll admit that I just assumed she was fine with allowing her son and daughter-in-law to clean and dress her after death. She had been in their care for a while, and everything between the three of them was loving and harmonious.

But as the time drew closer to Emma's death, she pulled me near to her and said, "You have to promise me that my son and daughter-in-law won't change me or dress me." I was shocked. There was no one else in place for that job, and time was of the essence. I panicked, but we managed to find someone else to dress her after death. And it was in the nick of time because Emma died that very night.

This is the kind of thing that needs to be planned well in advance, and we must make sure the person we designate is comfortable with the job, because it is indeed a very personal one. If someone is squeamish about it, they will be in a difficult position at the worst time for them, and the goal, of course, is to make the death experience as positive as it can possibly be for everyone involved.

Environment is also very important. Think about how your environment affects you every day. If you're surrounded by dirt and clutter, it impacts your mood. When the environment around a dying person is conducive to peace and calm, it helps facilitate a good death for them and everyone around them. Of course, don't get so busy cleaning that you exhaust yourself or fail to spend quality time with your loved one while you can. Just be aware of their environment, and do what's feasible to make it comfortable for them and for you.

With these issues in mind, ask your loved one these questions with regard to physical end-of-life care:

Questions with regard to **where**

1. Where would you like to be cared for at the end of life? (Refer back to the options mentioned in chapter 2.)

_____

_____

_____

2. If you want to be cared for at home, as is true for most people, what would you need to do now to make that happen? (Refer back to chapter 2. You might need to work further on this answer in the Financial Good Death chapter.)

_____

_____

_____

3. If you could not be cared for at home and needed to be in a care facility, do you know of one that would be acceptable to you? (If not, now is the time to research these facilities and find out what would be feasible.)

_____

_____

_____

Questions with regard to **who**

1. Who do you want to care for you at the end of life?

_____

2. Who would you feel most comfortable having as your physical caretaker for bathing and changing your clothes at the end of life?

_____

3. If your first choice for bathing and changing your clothes is not possible, who would be your second choice?

_____

Questions with regard to your environment

1. What would you like your surroundings to look like at the end of your life?

_____

_____

_____

2. How do you want your surroundings to smell? Do you want aromatherapy or candles?

_____

_____

_____

3. How do you want your surroundings to sound? Is there specific music that you like, or would you prefer ocean or other nature sounds?

_____

_____

_____

4. How do you want your environment to feel? Do you want it to be quiet and spiritual, or would you prefer people be talkative and jovial?

_____

_____

_____

5. Would you like to be provided with warm blankets if you're cold?

_____

6. Animals are often very important to people, so please specify if you want pets to be a part of your end-of-life care family. Or perhaps you would love a visit from a friend's pet or a trained emotional support animal.

_____

_____

_____

Questions with regard to personal care

1. Do you have a preference for personal grooming? Would you like your hair and nails done, and if so, who should do this task for you? Would you like to wear particular clothing?

_____

_____

_____

2. How comfortable do you want to be? If you have pain, on a scale from 1 to 10, with 10 being the most pain you could possibly feel, at which number would you like to be kept?

_____

_____

_____

3. Do you want any holistic therapies? These might include Reiki healing, massage, therapeutic touch, and aromatherapy, among others. Please specify.

_____

_____

_____

4. How do you want people to physically interact with you? What do you need in terms of the way others interact physically with you in order to feel that you have your dignity and that you are respected?

_____

_____

_____

_____

CHOICES FOR THE SACRED VIGIL PERIOD

The vigil period is the time right before someone dies. It usually lasts anywhere from three days to just a few hours. During this time, the dying person is usually in a deep sleep coma, but they can still hear.

Some of the following questions are similar to the ones in the

Choices for End-of-Life Care section above, but your loved one may want to make some different choices for the vigil period.

1. Who do you want to be present with you at the time of your death?

_____

_____

_____

2. How do you want your surroundings to look?

_____

_____

_____

3. How do you want your surroundings to smell? Do you want aromatherapy or candles?

_____

_____

_____

4. How do you want your surroundings to sound? You might want a very specific song to be played at this time, or you might like ocean or other nature sounds.

_____

_____

_____

5. How do you want your environment to feel? Do you want it to be quiet and spiritual, or would you prefer people be talkative and jovial?

_____

_____

_____

6. Do you have any special rituals you want to implement at the time of death?

_____

_____

_____

7. Are there any special readings or prayers you would like to be shared during the vigil period?

_____

_____

_____

8. Would you like family and loved ones to share stories of how you touched their lives throughout your lifetime?

_____

_____

_____

9. What are the most important things you want people to know about this moment? Do you have any special requests?

_____

_____

_____

CHOICES FOR IMMEDIATELY AFTER DEATH

I strongly recommend that people choose to have a viewing after death, but this is, of course, very much a matter of personal or cultural preference. Some religions, like Judaism, do not have a viewing.

1. How long do you want to stay at home after the time of death?

_____

2. Do you want a viewing? If so, how do you want it to be done?

_____

_____

_____

3. Lovingly bathing and dressing a loved one is an incredibly special and empowering experience. If you would like this, who would

you like to perform this task? Choose two people, as two are usually required to handle the body of someone who is deceased.

_____

_____

4. How would you like to be dressed? Choose an outfit that you love if that's in keeping with your religious traditions. Some people prefer a plain, natural shroud.

_____

_____

_____

5. How would you like to look in terms of hair, makeup, nails, and perhaps scent? You might like someone to wash and style your hair or apply your favorite nail color, perfume, or aftershave.

_____

_____

_____

CHOICES FOR THE FUNERAL/LIFE CELEBRATION/ MEMORIAL

1. What kind of funeral, life celebration, or memorial would you like, and where would you like it to be held? Include if you would like a viewing, or if you prefer a closed casket or no casket.

_____

_____

_____

If you wish to have a funeral/wake and a separate memorial service or life celebration, answer the following questions for each.

2. Who do you want to be invited?

_____

_____

_____

3. Would you like flowers? If so, what type?

_____

_____

_____

4. Would you like silk drapes to decorate the casket, or would you like to decorate it in some other way?

_____

_____

_____

5. Would you like photos to be displayed? If so, are there any special photos you want to include? Would you like a slideshow to be shown?

_____

_____

_____

6. Would you like special readings, prayers, or poems to be read? If so, who would you like to read them?

_____

_____

_____

7. Would you like specific music to be played? If so, what music? Would you like it to be recorded or played live? If the latter, who would you like to play or sing?

_____

_____

_____

8. Who would you like to write your eulogy? Do you want to write your own or have more than one eulogy read?

_____

_____

_____

9. Would you like food to be served, and if so, what kind of food? Are there specific recipes you would like to be included?

_____

_____

_____

10. Would you like to have a FUNeral like Shatzi's that I told you about in chapter 6?

_____

11. Do you want to plan a living wake before you are incapacitated?

_____

12. If you want to plan a living wake, answer questions 2, 3, 4, 5, 6, 7, and 9 for this event.

_____

_____

_____

_____

_____

_____

_____

_____

_____

_____

_____

_____

CHOICES ABOUT DISPOSITION OF THE BODY

Review chapter 7 for the different kinds of burials and cremation, and ask your loved one to specify their preferences.

1. Do you want a standard funeral with or without embalming, a green/natural burial, a fire cremation, a water/aqua cremation, or human composting?

_____

2. Where would you like to be buried?

_____

3. If you want a casket, what kind of casket do you want?

_____

4. Do you want to do a body donation or donate organs?

_____

CHOICES ABOUT ONGOING HONORING

Grief doesn't end after two weeks. We never stop missing the ones we love, and we don't have to. Commemorating the love they brought to our lives on a regular basis not only is beautiful, but allows our grief to shift into a healthy honoring and helps us recognize that their love is always available to us.

With that in mind, I recommend asking your loved one how and when they would like to be honored after they're gone. Be specific, and make it personal and joyful.

1. When would you like to be honored after you're gone? On birthdays, anniversaries, or other special days?

_____

_____

_____

2. Is there anything in particular you would like your loved ones to do when you are remembered and commemorated?

_____

_____

_____

PEACE OF MIND

When your loved one chooses what they want for the end of their life, it's a gift not only to themselves, but to their family and friends. As my student Rachel Thompson said, "When my mom got pancreatic cancer, it was devastating for me and my two brothers, but because she had chosen every detail for her end-of-life care (even paying for her burial plot ahead of time), the experience was so much easier."

And as Leo showed us, the choices people make at the end of life can be empowering and give them a sense of control. These choices can allow them to have the highest quality of life every day, even up to their last day. When people shared how happy and at peace Leo was, their sadness was transformed to awe and gratitude.

While everyone must make their own decision with regard to treatment options, it's telling that Leo lived two months longer than Rick. Whatever choices someone makes, a physical good death requires intentionality and a conscious effort to answer the right questions and plan appropriately. When people are attuned to their individual needs and wants, they can craft an end-of-life story that brings peace of mind to everyone involved during such a challenging time.

9

A Mental Good Death

> If we wish to die well, we must learn how to
> live well: Hoping for a peaceful death, we
> must cultivate peace in our mind, and in our
> way of life.
>
> —Dalai Lama

find that the way most people think about death is based on their
first experience of it. It's like the imprinting of baby ducks, who
will follow the first person they see after they're born. Whatever
that first experience may be sets the tone for how we relate to death
for the rest of our life unless something significant changes it.

So take a moment to think back to your first memory of death.
For most of us, it was a grandparent, pet, or wild animal. In my
case, it was a baby bird that fell from its nest. Or it might have been
through an animated film like *Bambi*, *The Lion King*, or *Finding
Nemo*. Or it might have been a parent, friend, or sibling for you.

How did you feel about it? How did the adults around you handle it? Did they grieve openly, or did they hide it from you? Were
you allowed to attend a funeral or prohibited from attending? Did
they try to pretend it was no big deal?

What do you remember being told about it? Did you feel fear, and do you think any current fears you have about death originated from this experience or perhaps a later one? Some people say, "I didn't know what happened to Grandma." A woman once told me she didn't even know her mother was sick until she came home from first grade one day to find her house full of people because her mother had died of cancer while she was at school. This purported protection of her only made it worse for her in the long run.

The way we *think* about death governs how we *feel* about it. If we think it's scary, we will feel scared. If we think it's a natural part of life that isn't to be feared, we won't be afraid. It's as simple as that, but also as complicated as our thoughts and feelings. If our early imprinting created fears within us, those fears can be tenacious. What we learn as children tends to stick to us like glue, and we have to consciously work to disengage from those early lessons.

I honestly think the dysfunction with regard to death that I have seen as a nurse and heard about from Doulagivers students around the globe is directly related to adults trying to shield and protect children from death. While their intentions are good, it tends to make children more afraid. I believe one of the greatest things we can do for our children is teach them that death is a natural part of life that happens to all living things.

Growing up, if you watched the adults around you ignore the reality of death and/or completely fall apart when they lost someone, it will color your own thinking and, in turn, your feelings—about both your own death and that of your loved ones. We'll discuss emotional peace of mind and an emotional good death in the next chapter. But in this chapter, we will talk about how we can change our *thinking* about death, which will also alter our emotional reaction to it.

This is a useful exercise for you as a caregiver who is faced with the death of a loved one, and if your loved one is open to discussing their experiences with it, the exercise can be beneficial for them as well. Of course, not everyone will be willing to talk about their history with the topic of death.

Before we go any further in our discussion of a mental good death and peace of mind, please answer the following questions about your early imprinting on the topic of death.

If your experience with death has been particularly difficult, take a deep breath and go at your own pace. Evaluating the origins of your fears may be the exact healing you need.

Journaling Exercise:
The Origins of Your Mental State About Death

1. Write down what you remember about your first experience with death.

_____

_____

_____

2. Do you recall anyone sitting you down and explaining it to you? If so, do you remember what was said? If not, what do you remember gleaning from their words or behaviors?

_____

_____

_____

3. Was that first experience mostly positive, or was it negative or frightening?

_____

4. How did the adults around you react to the death?

_____

_____

_____

5. Looking back from an adult perspective, do you think that first experience and/or the way you saw adults reacting has influenced the way you perceive death now?

_____

_____

_____

6. If you extracted that influence, what might you feel about death instead?

_____

_____

_____

7. Have you ever seen someone who was dying? What was the experience like?

_____

_____

_____

8. Have you ever seen a dead body? What was the experience like?

_____

_____

_____

9. Have you heard stories of negative end-of-life experiences?

_____

10. Have you heard stories of peaceful end-of-life experiences?

_____

11. Have those experiences altered your thinking about death, and has it been positive or negative?

_____

_____

_____

12. Do you have family members or friends who won't allow you to discuss end-of-life plans, and has that affected your mental state of mind about death?

_____

_____

_____

13. Are you concerned about what happens after death, and do your religious beliefs make you worry whether you will go to a good place?

_____

_____

_____

14. Do you feel you need to make some amends in order to feel better about what will happen to you after death?

_____

15. Do you worry that you haven't done everything you have wanted to do, and can you make peace with that?

_____

16. Can you imagine accepting death?

_____

I'm aware that these might seem like heavy and difficult questions, but answering them can greatly help you begin to unravel why you think about death the way you do. And if you think of it negatively, it just might be that this thinking isn't rational or based on anything that needs to be lasting. In other words, you can change the way you think about death, and that's one of the main points of this book.

You may also find that you can't pinpoint the origin of your fear of death. Many times, when I've worked with a caregiver or terminally ill patient with a great deal of fear about death, we can't point to a particular relationship or moment in time. Sometimes it just seems to be fear of the unknown, which is understandable, but that fear can be dissipated and eased when we come to a place of acceptance.

You might also want to think about the "death imprinting" that happens to the children around you. How can you facilitate a more peaceful first experience of death for them?

THE FIVE STAGES OF GRIEF

During my time as a hospice and oncology nurse, life was often confusing and frustrating. I sought direction and clarity wherever I could. Even though she died in 2004, Dr. Elisabeth Kübler-Ross was and remains a guiding force in my work. Her relentless tenacity to educate and bring healing to the world continues to encourage me to be the voice of the voiceless. She was instrumental in my decision to provide free education and resources to others and to help reduce the fear of death by bringing back its sacredness.

Dr. Kübler-Ross was a Swiss-American psychiatrist and author recognized for her pioneering work in the field of thanatology (the study of death and dying). In the late 1960s, she began interviewing terminally ill patients, seeking to understand their experiences and needs. This led to her development of the Five Stages of Grief, which she detailed in her groundbreaking 1969 book, *On Death and Dying*. These stages have been widely adopted in counseling and psychology.

The Five Stages of Grief don't necessarily happen to us in any particular order, and we may not go through all of them. We also may start to experience them as soon as someone receives a terminal diagnosis, long before death occurs, and the dying person goes through these as well. They are:

1. **Denial:** While your experience may be different, this is often the first reaction to loss. It is a common defense mechanism that numbs the intensity of our overwhelming emotions. In this stage, we might believe the diagnosis is somehow mistaken, or we might struggle to accept that our loved one is gone.

2. **Anger:** As the reality of the loss sets in, frustration and anger often follow. It might be directed at ourselves, others, God, or even the person who is dying or has died. We might feel abandoned, even though we know the person we have lost is not to blame.

3. **Bargaining:** During this stage, we think about what might have been done to prevent the loss, such as "If only we had gotten medical help sooner..." It's our way of dealing with the feelings of helplessness that accompany loss.

4. **Depression:** This stage involves feelings of sadness, regret, fear, and uncertainty. We might become quiet, refuse visitors, and spend much of our time crying and grieving. It's a time to truly sit with our emotions.

5. **Acceptance:** Acceptance doesn't mean that we are ever fine with the loss or that grief is completely done. It just means that we have come to accept the reality of it. This stage brings us more emotional stability and a return to our regular daily activities.

These stages are very similar to the Doulagivers three phases of end of life that we discussed in chapter 3: shock, stabilization, and transition. Yes, they are emotional, but moving through them is what helps us reach a place of mental peace of mind and acceptance.

While Dr. Kübler-Ross never specifically used the term "mental good death," she did discuss the concept of a "good death." For her, it's one in which the person has accepted their mortality and can face their end without fear or anxiety. That's the true meaning of acceptance and mental peace of mind.

With all the beautiful work that she did for a good death

education, did Dr. Kübler-Ross have a good death herself? In 1994, a fire destroyed her house in Virginia, where she had plans to build a home and AIDS hospice for abandoned babies. AIDS was still relatively new, and there was a great deal of fear about it. Soon after the loss of her home, however, she suffered a series of strokes that left her compromised for the last nine years of her life. Her son, Ken, who now serves as the president of the Elisabeth Kübler-Ross Foundation and generously shared this story with me, cared for his mother in Arizona for much of this time until she finally went into a nursing home for the last two years of her journey.

During the nine-year period, Dr. Kübler-Ross often declared, "I'm ready to die" and would even call Ken to say, "Don't make plans for next Tuesday, as that is the day I'm going to die."

She had always said, "Once you learn your lessons, you can graduate." But she was angry. Due to her strokes, she was dependent on others to care for her, which is something she absolutely hated. Ken says that his mother's last lesson was to learn to give up control and allow herself to receive love and care from others. As soon as she learned this lesson, as evidenced by the happiness and joy she showed while in her nursing home, she was able to finally graduate in complete peace, surrounded by those who loved her. She reached a place of "radical acceptance." Let's talk about what that means.

RADICAL ACCEPTANCE

Radical acceptance is associated with Dialectical Behavioral Therapy (DBT) and is based on the idea that even when we don't have the power to change our current reality, we do have the power to change our attitude (our mind) about it. We stop bargaining, we stop fighting it, and we surrender to what is true, making peace with it. After all, every single one of us is touched by death at some point—first the death of others and, finally, our own death.

All of the work you and your loved one are doing throughout this book can make grief easier, whether it's the anticipatory grief that comes with knowing death is imminent or the grief that happens after death. I have witnessed this with countless people. Learning about end of life, planning ahead, and having support soften the blow and facilitate radical acceptance.

This acceptance is the cornerstone of mental peace of mind and a mental good death. That doesn't mean I want you to chastise yourself or judge your loved one for continuing to have fears and worries. Radical acceptance means accepting those emotions as well. They are a normal human part of this process. You don't have to be perfect in your radical acceptance. I only suggest that you and your loved one strive for it as a way to ease the pain of dealing with death. So be gentle with yourself and the dying at all times.

Think of radical acceptance as letting go of resistance. Buddhists call it "accepting what is." How often in our lives do we resist what we can't change, complaining to the point of exhaustion? It causes us stress, struggle, and emotional turmoil. Think of that Alcoholics Anonymous prayer: "God grant me the serenity to accept the things I cannot change, the courage to change the things I can, and the wisdom to know the difference." When we can reach this place in relation to death, it's easier to take care of practical matters, make sound decisions, and be fully present with our loved ones in the precious moments at end of life. It allows us to move forward without getting stuck. We can then relish those last moments in their sacredness and experience them with a combination of joy and sadness rather than with pain alone.

So how do you and your loved one arrive at a place of radical acceptance and mental peace of mind?

- Start by focusing on the present moment as much as you can. Remind yourself that you can't change the past or predict the future. But you can be *here right now* and experience each moment fully with the people you love. You can live each day like its own "one little lifetime" with a heightened level of appreciation and not waiting for "someday."

- One easy way to ground yourself in the present is to say three things aloud that you feel grateful for in your life right now, and it will shift your energy instantly to the moment.

- Acknowledge what you feel, including your fears and immense grief. Allow yourself to feel them and let them pass through like visitors or waves that you surf until calm seas come again. Try not to grasp them and hold them because that only causes them to fester.

- Strive to let go of judgments and criticisms of yourself and others.

- Embrace the situation as the opportunity for growth and learning that it is.

- Learn mindfulness techniques, and practice quiet meditation to calm your nervous system and bring yourself an experience of peace.

- Remember the most valuable moments you shared with your loved one during their life. Appreciate those moments with gratitude and, to the degree you can, embrace the love you have shared and the sacredness of this cycle of life and death that we all share.

- As you recall the entire end-of-life experience, try to reframe it by creating a "highlight reel" in your mind that replays the positive moments.

- Understand that many times, the depth and level of our grief is directly related to the amount of love and connection we had with the person we lost. While we'll no longer have that person in our life in physical form, we will always have the love, experiences, and memories they brought to our life.

- Remember that there is no right or wrong way to grieve. Besides meditation, try taking walks in nature, spending time with the people you love, and engaging in forms of dance/movement. Give yourself the self-care you need physically, emotionally, and spiritually, all of which will help you find radical acceptance and mental peace of mind.

See Appendix A at the back of the book for information about prolonged grief disorder, Appendix B for what to say to someone who's grieving, and Appendix C for a quick and handy checklist for healing from grief.

In the next chapter, we'll talk about how to achieve emotional peace of mind, which, of course, is closely related to mental peace of mind.

10

An Emotional Good Death

What we once enjoyed and deeply loved we
can never lose, for all that we love deeply
becomes part of us.

—Helen Keller

t started like any morning. I was doing my rounds in the oncology
unit as usual, and most patients were still sleeping or just wak-
ing up—also as usual. But when I entered Mrs. Garner's room,
I found her crying and sobbing in relentless pain. The situation was
so severe that several case managers and social workers were present,
trying to resolve the situation for her, as her husband stood by in a
state of helplessness and fright.

When I looked at Mrs. Garner's records, I saw that she was
receiving enough pain medicine to put a horse into a palliative coma.
"How is it possible that she's still suffering so much?" I thought. I'm
sure the white coats in the room were wondering the same thing.

So what was going on? The truth is that there are times in the
end-of-life journey when someone's emotional pain is so intense that
it presents as physical pain. This means that we can throw as much
narcotic pain medication at it as we want, but the meds won't make

a dent in the pain. Cases like Mrs. Garner's helped me understand that when a patient's pain isn't helped by a good pain management regimen, it's time to look for the emotional cause.

At the end of life, all of the patient's feelings, emotions, trauma, and/or baggage bubble to the top, and it can feel overwhelming to process. It's as though all of it wants to be resolved before they take flight beyond this world, which would provide them with a final opportunity to clear the air. When someone can indeed find a degree of peace in this way at the end of life, it is a gift not only to them but also to the ones they leave behind.

Of course, this healing can happen only if someone is willing. None of us can "fix" anyone else's emotional pain. It's their journey, not ours, and we can't push anyone into emotional spaces they aren't ready to inhabit. Nevertheless, one of the most effective tools to help someone resolve emotional issues is to provide a safe, unconditionally loving space that can cushion them enough to *choose* to go there.

There are three main categories of emotional pain that most people confront at the end of life:

1. **Regrets** for what they have done and for what they haven't done
2. **Trauma** from the past that has kept them stuck, sad, or depressed
3. **Lack of forgiveness** toward others and toward themselves

Let's explore each of these categories separately.

REGRETS

I know they say death is the number one fear in the world. But having been privileged to be with many, many people at the end of life, my experience has shown that the fear of death itself isn't the main issue for most. It's the regrets.

When we live life without acknowledging that death will one day be a natural part of our journey, treating it as if it's optional, we don't take care of many of the important things we are meant to do, learn, and be. We put end-of-life plans out of our mind entirely, or we tell ourselves, "I'll get to it eventually…when I retire" or "when I have enough money" or "when the time is right." Yet time is the most precious commodity we have, especially since none of us knows how much of it we will ultimately have.

Once we know for sure that our time is limited, the regrets come bubbling to the surface. I have heard hundreds of "deathbed regret confessions," and I have seen commonalities and patterns among them. From my experience, here are the top four regrets that have been shared with me.

Regret #1: I regret not following my heart guidance and aligning with my true purpose.

From the first day of our lives, we are influenced by and conditioned to believe what society and our family believe. We are taught to follow the thinking of our ego and rational mind, making choices from that place about our career, our relationships, and how we present ourselves.

We tell ourselves that even though we hate our career choice, it will bring us a good income. Even if we have reservations about our romantic partner, they look right on paper. We tell ourselves that we have to dress and look a certain way in order to be accepted. But we are not just human *doings;* we are primarily human *beings.* As such, the guidance of our heart's higher wisdom is also available to us, yet many of us fail to make choices based on that wisdom, even though it can be much better at guiding us toward the things that bring meaning and fulfillment to our lives. Instead, far too many of us lead lives that keep us feeling unhappy, stuck, and lost.

Deep down, we all know we are here for a reason and a purpose. When we follow our higher wisdom, we can align with that purpose and experience a deeper connection to this life we've been given. Understanding that we have two separate guidance systems can change everything.

Regret #2: I regret not having the courage to love others fully.

One of my patients was a sixty-nine-year-old man who had obtained incredible wealth and success. He was among the top 1 percent of income earners in the US. He had houses everywhere, a private plane, and more cars than anyone could possibly drive. On his deathbed, he talked about all the family and friends with whom he had cut ties over money, jealousy, and petty arguments. "I held on to anger and cut people off for stupid things, and I can't even remember why. At the time, I thought it was easier, but I ended up sad, lonely, and alone for most of my life. I never found love. I never gave myself the chance to experience it, and now I know this is the entire point of life. I get it now! Please tell others my story."

As a young hospice nurse, I was struck by this regret, which I heard from diverse people from all religions and cultures. *Love* was the main wisdom they repeated as they neared their transition. *It is the key, the answer, and the medicine.*

Regret #3: I regret not having the courage to let others love me fully.

Due to the hurt and pain we experience in life, it's very common to build walls around our heart in an effort to protect it. This can be healthy in the short term, but when we build walls continuously over time and never take them down, we end up building a fortress. No love gets in, and no love gets out. We may think this practice keeps us safe, but we're actually in a prison of our own making.

When people reach the end of life, they regret that prison they built and wish they had shown more courage to open their heart and let others in.

Regret #4: I regret that I judged myself so much and didn't love myself more.

If love is the key, the answer, and the medicine, unconditional self-love is the foundation of that. Learning to love ourselves without conditions is what allows us to open our hearts to loving others as we allow others to love us. If the meaning of life is to experience true, unconditional love, that love has to start with us.

When I work with people at the end of life and they share their regrets, I suggest they go back to the time of each regret and remember all of the details. I ask them the following questions: *What was your job? Where did you live? Who was in your life? What struggles or challenges were you experiencing?* Then I ask them this: *Considering where you were and what you were going through, were you doing the best you could?* The answer is almost always yes!

It's amazing how little empathy we have for ourselves. When we understand that life is a learning experience and that it can be very hard, we can see that the choices we made at certain times in our lives were the best we could make under those circumstances. This awareness allows us to find peace and have compassion for ourselves, which allows us to come to terms with our past regrets.

TRAUMA

Emotional trauma is a deeply distressing experience that overwhelms our ability to cope. It can result from a single event, a series of events, or ongoing stress. It can shake our sense of security, making us feel helpless and vulnerable in a world that feels dangerous. And emotional trauma is a part of the human experience; we all have it. Here are key points about emotional trauma:

- It often stems from situations in which we feel powerless.
- It can originate from natural disasters, violent attacks, the loss of loved ones, or witnessing a horrific event.
- It can lead to severe anxiety, depression, panic attacks, and post-traumatic stress disorder (PTSD).
- It can manifest physically as headaches, fatigue, sleep disturbances, disease, and changes in appetite.

The key is learning to process and/or heal our trauma so that it doesn't keep us from living a beautiful and full life or having a peaceful and sacred death. This usually requires therapy and a commitment to feeling better. It can take time, and it can be painful. But it paves the way for emotional relief and freedom in the long term.

When someone reaches the end of life, they may no longer have the time to fully heal their trauma, but when they can surrender to self-compassion, self-love, and the self-forgiveness I will discuss in the next section, they can heal a great deal of their trauma in their last months, weeks, or moments. As caregivers, we can help facilitate this healing for them by being as compassionate and forgiving as possible.

FORGIVENESS

I knew a twenty-six-year-old woman named Allie in New York City who had a promising career in the fashion industry and a great group of friends. One day, she received a phone call from her aunt, telling her that her estranged father was dying in England and wanted to see her before he died. At first, Allie thought, "No way!" In fact, she couldn't believe his audacity, since he hadn't been there for her during her entire life. But after a few days, she reluctantly decided to go see him.

As Allie walked into her father's hospital room, she found him surrounded by a luminous aura unlike anything she had ever seen before. Enthusiastically, he said to her, "Please forgive me. I forgive you. I love you! Everything is okay." She was taken aback, but the love and positive energy emanating from her father in that moment healed her heart, and she's so glad she made that trip. After twenty-six years of pain, hurt, and resentment, it gave her a kind of loving closure she hadn't dreamed was possible.

Forgiveness is the single greatest transformational tool at the end of life (or at any time during life). I can honestly say that the most beautiful end-of-life experiences I have witnessed have been because the person surrendered to the power of forgiveness before they died. (This is part of the stabilization phase, as I mentioned in chapter 3.)

So often, I have watched forgiveness clear the dying person's guilt, clear the guilt of others, and wipe the slate clean. It "cleans" the energy of the person who is dying and anyone else around them who is open to that experience.

Unfortunately, many people brush off forgiveness because they misunderstand it. I have heard numerous people say, "They don't deserve to be forgiven." But forgiveness is a deliberate decision to release feelings of resentment or vengeance toward someone who has harmed us, *regardless of whether they deserve that forgiveness.* The act of forgiving is for *us,* not for them. It doesn't mean we forget or condone an offense, nor does it mean we absolve someone of the consequences of their actions.

As Allie discovered, no matter how close we feel we are to someone or how much we think we know about someone, we never know the whole story. So when we want to forgive someone, it's helpful to remember that everyone is carrying burdens we know nothing about. This can help us transform our anger into empathy.

Holding on to resentment takes so much of our energy. As they say, staying angry with someone is like giving them free real estate in our mind or like drinking poison and expecting the other person to die. Just as my wealthy patient did, we regret holding on to grudges when we reach end of life. We realize the futility of it and wish we had realized that futility sooner. Forgiveness is simply an act of releasing ourselves from the energy-draining attachment to the person or experience that hurt us. It sets us free.

It's also true that as caregivers and loved ones of someone who is at end of life, when we feel we can genuinely offer them our forgiveness, it's a tremendous gift to them—but perhaps even more so to ourselves.

SELF-FORGIVENESS

People usually find that it's easier to forgive others than it is to forgive themselves. We tend to hold ourselves to a more stringent standard than we hold others, so we're hypercritical of our mistakes. It helps to revisit the questions I ask patients about regrets. When someone realizes they did the best they could in the moment, they can begin to forgive themselves for their imperfections. After all, perfection is impossible.

When we come from a place of heart-centered love and compassion, it's much easier to forgive ourselves or someone else.

The Role Unforgiveness Plays in Illness

Both Johns Hopkins Hospital and Harvard Medical School, as well as other prestigious medical institutions, have published articles about the effects of unforgiveness on our physical health, as well as emotional and mental health. You probably wouldn't be surprised to learn that studies have linked forgiveness with reduced stress, anxiety, and depression, as well as improved sleep. But it has also been linked to lowering our heart attack risk, physical pain, blood pressure, and cholesterol. This happens because chronic anger puts the body in fight-or-flight mode, which activates a lot of stress-related physical responses that can turn into chronic conditions or even disease.[1]

How do we know we are suffering from unforgiveness? Here are the main signs and symptoms:

- Hurt
- Anger and resentment
- Guilt
- Depression
- Feeling unloved
- Self-sabotaging behavior
- Recurring memories that cause anger, guilt, or shame
- Emotional, mental, and/or physical pain

What End-of-Life Patients Say About Forgiveness

First and foremost, they say, "Do not wait!" We spoke earlier in the chapter about regrets, and unforgiveness is one of the main regrets that people have at end of life. This is a sacred time in which the dying person may change their perspective significantly. Often, they suddenly see their life through an entirely different lens.

I call it a lens of love. It offers them a window of opportunity to see their life challenges and experiences as lessons for growth. In doing so, they often let go of victim mentality.

In 2019, I was able to present Doulagivers trainings all over the beautiful country of Thailand. One of my last events was at a temple that took care of people who were dying from serious illnesses. The temple had a four-pillar approach that included meditation, a plant-based diet, yoga, and forgiveness.

There was a thirty-one-year-old man there who was dying of pancreatic cancer. He had felt anger toward his father for most of his life, but he found freedom in his last months through the forgiveness practice at the temple. I witnessed others there having similar experiences. I will never forget the bright smiles on the faces of these people. It was as if they no longer had a care in the world despite the fact that they were within months of the end of their lives.

Allie and her estranged father experienced forgiveness in a profound way as well. Of course, I know that relationships are complicated, and people have to be willing to enter that window of opportunity. But there is no better time than the end of life to have these conversations.

As Allie's father learned to say similar words, I recommend saying the following to achieve emotional peace, as I mentioned in chapter 3. This can be said by or to the dying person depending on the choices of the people involved, but I have found these statements to be simple and often all-encompassing:

> I forgive you.
> Please forgive me.
> I love you.
> Thank you.
> I wish you only peace.

EMOTIONAL PEACE OF MIND PLANNER

Emotional peace of mind is the result of having done our work to heal emotional trauma, regrets, and unforgiveness. It isn't easy. It takes courage and strength to confront our emotional pain in order to shine light on it. But once this is done, the energy is neutralized and transmuted. Only the light can remain.

By the time we reach end of life, our time to resolve all of these issues is limited, so the earlier someone can begin this part of the process, the better. But emotional peace of mind can be achieved even when someone has little time left on this earth, and as caregivers or loved ones, we can help facilitate this aspect of peace of mind for the dying, as well as for ourselves.

The following Emotional Peace of Mind Planner is divided into three sections:

1. Unresolved issues
2. Trauma
3. Forgiveness

Unresolved Issues
Which people and experiences in your current life or past evoke feelings of anger, guilt, shame, or emotional pain for you? Write down each one and the emotions you associate with each.

_____

_____

_____

_____

_____

_____

_____

_____

_____

_____

For each person and experience on your list, answer these questions:

1. What is the truth in this situation?

_____

_____

_____

2. What were the other people involved experiencing in their life at that time?

_____

_____

_____

3. If I regret my behavior in the situation, what was happening in my life at the time that led to my behavior?

_____

_____

_____

If possible, please take your time with this, and allow yourself the love and space to work through it slowly.

Trauma

Whether we are conscious of it or not, our trauma can be a time bomb waiting to explode, and it bleeds out in our resentments and behaviors toward others. Sometimes, we make assumptions based on our past traumas. For example, we may automatically believe others are untrustworthy because we have been betrayed.

Think of emotional trauma as a photograph of a feeling captured in time, which remains locked in that same emotional state until we do the work to heal it. When something happens to activate the trauma, it can be very painful and intense. So what can someone do to heal it, especially if they're at the end of life?

1. Life review. Get a notebook and ask your loved one to write down the main experiences they remember. If they can't write them, you can do it for them or make a recording of their memories. This is called a life review. This exercise is bound to bring up some discomfort, but that isn't a bad thing. Allowing ourselves to feel the discomfort, possibly anger or hurt, is where the healing begins. That's where a shift in the trauma happens. If you are facilitating a loved one through this exercise, remind them that they are courageous, supported, and loved. Most people have an internal "highlight reel" of their life, so their life review doesn't have to be extensive or long. But don't rush your loved one through it. Allow them to tell their story, which, in and of itself, is healing. You may learn some cherished information in the process that helps you understand them better. If they struggle to get started, ask questions like the ones that follow. There are a lot of potential questions here, however, so you might want to do the life review in increments. It can be a great way to have quality conversations with each other during this last period of time together, and it can bring up wonderful memories as well as traumatic events for healing.

- Where did you grow up?
- Did you ever have a nickname?
- How many siblings did/do you have? Tell me about them.
- What do you remember most about your parents, grandparents, or early caregivers?

- What other family members do you especially remember?
- What was your favorite subject in school?
- What teacher do you remember most?
- Tell me about your favorite activities when you were a kid.
- Talk about the houses or apartments where you've lived throughout your life.
- Have you ever collected anything?
- Who has been your greatest friend in life, and what are/were they like?
- What was your first job?
- When did you first fall in love?
- What was it like when you met your spouse(s)?
- Tell me about your wedding(s).
- Tell me about your child(ren).
- What's your favorite memory from your career?
- What or who was the hardest loss of your life?
- Have you ever experienced a crime or serious accident?
- What makes you laugh the most?
- What's your favorite color, food, song, movie, and book?
- Where have you traveled?
- What's the hardest choice you've ever had to make?
- What's the best decision you ever made?
- What's the scariest thing that ever happened to you?
- What do you feel is your greatest accomplishment or greatest source of pride?
- Have you had any beloved pets?

- If you had to choose the most memorable moment of your life, what would it be?
- What are you most grateful for?

2. Exercise to release trauma. In order to be healed and released, emotional trauma must be felt, seen, heard, honored, and witnessed. Once it is validated, it will transform, and healing can occur. With that goal in mind, suggest your loved one spend twenty minutes each day, if possible, to simply sit with their feelings as they read through or recall their life review. Ask them to observe the sensations and emotions in their body. These will intensify as they focus on them. Some of the feelings may be just as intense as they were when they first felt them, perhaps many years ago. The goal is to be with their feelings, to fully be with themselves. If they would like, they can repeat this sentence like a mantra: "I am completely safe now and own my personal power." Of course, if your loved one is very frail, it may not be possible for them to do this extensively.

3. The inner child. If your loved one finds themselves experiencing an emotionally traumatic memory, suggest they observe the memory from as objective a perspective as they can, and try altering it mentally in a way that feels emotionally positive. This is what psychologists call "inner child work." If they find themselves witnessing a traumatic childhood memory, for example, this is their opportunity to offer themselves the care they didn't receive at the time. As they do, they can connect with the small child inside of them (we all have one), hold that child, and give that child the love, safety, and reassurance they need and perhaps didn't receive at the time of the trauma.

Forgiveness: The Path to Unconditional Love

1. Your forgiveness list. Ask your loved one to make a list of all the people they need to forgive and all the things they would like to be forgiven for. (You may choose to do this and some of the other exercises in this chapter for yourself as well.)

2. Techniques to forgive. If they struggle to forgive someone or themselves, they can try these steps:

(a) Picture the person (or yourself) as a small child, and then work on forgiving them.

(b) Feel as much empathy and compassion for them (or yourself) as you can.

(c) Ask yourself: Were they (or you) doing the best they (or you) could at the time?

(d) Remind yourself that their actions might stem from a place of hurt and anger you know nothing about.

(e) Remember that forgiveness doesn't mean you condone what happened, forget what happened, have to tell the other person you forgive them, or allow the other person into your life again. *Forgiveness is for you!*

11

A Financial Good Death

Only put off until tomorrow what you are
willing to die having left undone.

—Pablo Picasso

Rachel and her two brothers were devastated when their
mother received a terminal stage 4 cancer diagnosis at the
age of fifty-eight. Doctors estimated that she wouldn't survive for longer than two or three months.

Unbeknownst to them, however, their mother, a former nurse,
had planned everything for her end of life. She had prepaid for her
funeral, casket, and burial plot. She created a living trust and transferred her assets to it so that Rachel and her brothers would have
access to the funds immediately without the need for probate. She
signed a last will and testament to cover anything in her estate that
she failed to cover in the trust.

"As hard as it was to say goodbye to Mom," Rachel says, "she
made it 90 percent easier on us by planning everything ahead of
time. I hate to think what it would have been like for us if we were
left to make decisions while so lost in grief."

Contrast that story with Dan and Carla. They were separated and living apart, but they were still legally married and shared a teenage daughter. One night, Dan came home from work, went to bed, and died of a heart attack in his sleep at age fifty-seven. Just like Rachel and her family, Carla and her daughter were utterly devastated.

But adding to their grief was the difficulty of figuring out Dan's accounts, getting into his cell phone, and finding his passwords for important websites. His papers were strewn all over his apartment, so it required painstakingly going through each piece to find what was important and needed. Dan also died without a will, which meant his estate, even though modest, was stuck in probate for more than a year. The stress and overwhelm all of this caused Carla and their daughter were immeasurable, and it was hardly what Dan wanted to leave for them.

These stories show the importance of financial peace of mind at end of life, for both the person who dies and the people they leave behind. Since most families don't plan in advance, far too many people are left to piece together accounts, passwords, and the wishes of the deceased. As a result, they often end up spending much more money than necessary.

It has broken my heart more times than I can remember to hear family members worry about how they were going to pay their loved one's hospital bill or about how a family member took expensive or sentimental items from the loved one's home without consulting other survivors. But this is what's likely to happen when we don't do any financial planning or designate who should get what.

When people do plan ahead, they can save their family and loved ones needless emotional upheaval, as well as thousands, if not tens of thousands, of dollars. Without the legal documents in place, settling an estate is a much more complicated matter, and it can get very ugly between family members as they fight over possessions. I have seen this kind of infighting go on for months or even years, as the grief becomes displaced by arguments over money. Families can even turn on each other over a single item.

Planning ahead, like Rachel's mother did, gives someone the peace of knowing their wishes are clear for their money and personal items. It gives those left behind the opportunity for a healthy and harmonious experience with grief, focusing on love rather than discord.

Unfortunately, despite the importance of estate planning, wills, and advance directives, more people seem to follow in Dan's footsteps. In fact, fewer people are planning ahead than they did in the past, according to an August 2023 analysis by the Center for Retirement Research at Boston College. In the ten years from 2008 to 2018, the share of households with someone over the age of seventy who had a will or trust went down from 70 percent to 63 percent. Another study by Caring.com has shown that the share of Americans over the age of fifty-five with a will reduced from 48 percent to 46 percent between 2020 and 2023. And people often blame procrastination for it.[1] This is not good news.

Sure, people get busy, and they don't want to think about death. But if they know about the potential consequences of putting it off, it's a nagging worry that they can alleviate simply by making up their mind to take care of it. If more people understood that it's unlikely to be as expensive or complex as they fear it will be, perhaps they would finally do it.

And trust me, the time to make financial decisions is *not* after someone receives a terminal diagnosis. This almost never goes well, if it even gets done at all in the midst of that kind of turmoil.

Imagine the stress of feeling terribly ill and trying to make decisions about your finances without the proper time or frame of mind to truly think about what you want. Financial decisions need to be well thought out, not done when someone is in a critical state.

This chapter is designed to take the guesswork out of it and show you the easiest and least expensive way to help your loved one attain financial peace of mind. I hope it will convince you that they can do it for far less money than you probably think, and that the great night's sleep everyone will get once these matters have been settled is worth whatever discomfort you all might feel during the process.

One caveat as I get ready to offer you advice: I'm not a lawyer, but I have done considerable research and spoken to attorneys and estate planning firms about what people need to do to prepare financially for end of life. Nevertheless, what you will read in this chapter should not be a substitute for legal advice, and the names of documents and specific steps to take vary greatly from one country to another.

LAST WILL AND TESTAMENT

A last will and testament is a legal document in which we express our wishes as to how possessions are to be distributed after our death, whether it's money, property, or personal items. The basics of this document are mostly the same throughout the world, although some of the terminology may differ. In the US, the deceased person in a will is the "testator," while the people who receive money, property, or goods are called "beneficiaries" or "inheritors." A "bequest" in a will is a gift given to a beneficiary. It can be money or most anything else. When a bequest is given to someone, it is "bequeathed" to them.

Of course, we usually think of it as the document that specifies the inheritance for our beneficiaries, who might be family members, friends, pets, and/or charities. But we can stipulate other things in a will as well, such as the kind of funeral or service we would like and where, as well as what should happen to our body after we die. We can name guardians for our children or pets, and we can specify how our debts and taxes will be paid.

The testator names an "executor" in the will, as well as an alternate executor in case the first person named cannot perform the necessary duties. When you are choosing an executor, make sure to ask them first. Do they have the time and inclination to deal with all the paperwork? The executor files the will with the probate court after the testator dies, which starts the probate process (more on that in a moment). (If you are a named executor, be sure to check with your state or country to see how much time you have to file the will after your loved one dies.)

What is probate? It's the legal process in the United States that establishes the validity and authenticity of someone's last will and testament after they die. Most every country has its own version of this.

The court where probate is done reviews the assets of the estate and determines what estate taxes, if any, must be paid to the government. States and countries vary as to whether probate is absolutely required, however. Some US states don't require it unless the estate is valued at a certain amount or higher.

Once the probate court gives the executor permission, it's their job to see that the testator's wishes are carried out and that the assets are distributed to the beneficiaries named in the will. It's also their job to pay estate taxes and any debts owed by the testator from the proceeds in the estate, as well as file a final income tax return on behalf of the estate. Note that the executor is not personally responsible for the taxes or debts of the deceased. Those monies come from the estate, which consists of the funds the testator left behind after their death. Sometimes there isn't enough money to cover all of a testator's debts, but if that happens, the executor is still not required to pay them.

When you or your loved one makes a will, be sure that any money left to beneficiaries actually exists in the estate. If the estate has less money than is listed in the will, it will delay probate and will be a lot more work for the executor, who will have to calculate the value of the estate before amounts to be given can be determined and distributed. Let's say your loved one wants to leave $10,000 to a grandchild. Make sure that amount exists in their accounts. Sometimes testators will leave specific amounts or items to certain people, while leaving the remainder of the estate to the spouse or children. If the spouse is the person named as a sole beneficiary in the will, the entire estate can be left to them. In that case, it isn't necessary to determine if there's enough money in the estate to cover the bequests.

Note, too, that if property is owned jointly, such as a house that's in the name of both spouses, it isn't included in the will. Instead, it immediately goes to the surviving spouse.

It's important to revisit our beneficiaries and executors regularly. Let's say someone made their will twenty years ago and named their then husband as executor, but they have since remarried and no longer speak to their ex-husband. Obviously, that needs to be changed right away!

When a person dies without a will, like Dan, they have died "intestate." The probate process is much more complicated in this case and gives control over to the probate court based on the laws of the particular state or country. In the US, if a person owns real estate in a different state from where they live, the laws of that state apply to what happens to the real estate. So dying intestate could mean more than one state's probate court obtains control over the assets. In other words, when we don't make our own decisions, they are made for us. This is the last thing anyone wants to happen, but many people procrastinate long enough that it's exactly what their family faces.

For one thing, the longer it takes for a will to complete probate, the more expensive it will be in terms of court costs. When we leave a will that is easy to authenticate, we can minimize those costs.

The good news is that in any US state, there are very few legal requirements for a will. You don't have to have a lawyer to make a will, and no state in the US requires that it be notarized. Famed singer Aretha Franklin wrote her will on a napkin. It wasn't witnessed, and it was later found in her couch. But the court deemed it as valid. When in doubt, just write it out!

Here are the legal requirements of a will in the United States to avoid disputes (check your country's requirements):

- The testator must know what property they have and what it means to leave it to someone after their death. Legally, this is called having "capacity" and is also known as being "of sound mind."

- The testator must create a document that names beneficiaries for at least some of their property.
- The testator must sign the document in the presence of two witnesses, who can be anyone.
- The document must also be signed by the two witnesses, who stipulate that they saw the testator sign the will and that the testator seemed to be of sound mind.

While it isn't necessary, it's helpful to add an affidavit (a document that you can find on the internet) in which the witnesses attest that they saw the testator sign the will. This extra document can help the will get through probate faster.

Certainly, if your loved one has the means to hire an attorney to handle the will and other documents mentioned in this chapter, that might be the option they choose. But it isn't necessary, and most of us can't afford the costs, nor do we have enough assets in our estate to merit such costs. I have spoken to lawyers, and they have all said it's perfectly fine to use online estate forms. You can also use online legal services for nominal fees. Of course, always check reviews before using such a service.

DOWNSIZING AND DECLUTTERING

Once someone has received a terminal diagnosis, it's too late to begin paring down their belongings. At that point, you want to care for them and spend as much time with them as you can. But if they start planning ahead early enough, they can think about what they really need to keep and what they can discard. In some European countries, this is a typical practice for people as early as age fifty. They begin to let go of items they won't need in order to make it easier for the people they leave behind. Weeding through a lot of stuff after someone dies is a tremendous amount of work, not to mention an emotional task.

While writing a last will and testament and thinking about what to bequeath to others, it might also be a good time to think about downsizing. Of course, it's best to avoid throwing things out and piling up our landfills more than necessary. So if someone else can use items like furniture or kitchen supplies, these things can be sold, given to a thrift shop, or advertised online to give away for free.

THE BENEFITS OF TRUSTS

In the US, a trust is a financial arrangement that allows a trustee or third party to hold assets owned by a grantor (sometimes called a trustor) for the benefit of a beneficiary or beneficiaries. I know that might sound like gibberish, so let's break it down. (Please check your country's laws and terms with regard to trusts.)

A grantor is a person (say, a parent) who has funds or property they want to give to a beneficiary (say, a child) at a particular time. When you buy a life insurance policy, for example, you specify a beneficiary or more than one beneficiary who will receive the value of the policy after your death. A beneficiary of a trust is the same.

A trustee is a person who is responsible for seeing that the beneficiary receives the assets named in the trust at the time specified. For example, a trustee might be the spouse or sibling of the parent in the above example. The trustee is literally someone who is trusted to hold the assets in their name until the time when the beneficiary is supposed to receive them.

Trusts can be arranged in a number of ways and can specify exactly how and when the assets pass to the beneficiaries. Trusts that are in effect while the grantor is still living are called living trusts. In this case, the grantor and the trustee can actually be the same person. The grantor just needs to name a substitute trustee in case they die or become incapacitated.

Let's look at an example to help you understand it. A grantor creates a trust for their underage children, and they don't want those children to receive the funds from the estate until they are twenty-one years old. If the grantor dies when the children are young, the trustee holds the funds for the estate and distributes them to the children when they come of age.

The main benefit of creating a trust is that it can often bypass the probate process. As a result, the beneficiaries can receive the funds without delay. Let's say I want to leave my entire estate to my son, but I want to avoid the costs of probate. I create a trust with myself as trustee and a chosen successor trustee (in case something happens to me) to distribute the funds to my son at the time I specify. I could also name myself as trustee with someone else as co-trustee to serve alongside me. If the trust sets forth that the funds go to my son after I die, the money would go to him immediately upon my death without the need to authenticate my will in the probate process. However, income from the funds in the trust is still subject to annual income taxes as long as I'm alive, and the funds are also still subject to estate taxes after I die.

You may have heard of both "revocable" and "irrevocable" trusts. A revocable trust is a document that can be changed by the grantor during their lifetime. It is flexible and can be dissolved at any time. An irrevocable trust *cannot* be changed once it has been signed, and a revocable trust becomes irrevocable once the grantor dies.

Why would anyone make an irrevocable trust if they can't change it? Well, the benefit of an irrevocable trust is that—because it can't be altered in the future—the funds are immediately transferred to the trust so that the grantor no longer has to pay taxes on the income generated by those funds on their personal income taxes, and it also minimizes estate taxes for the beneficiary. (Since a revocable trust can be altered, the funds aren't transferred until the moment the trust becomes irrevocable, or upon the grantor's death.) So a grantor might choose this option if their primary aim is to reduce taxes while they are still alive and estate taxes after they have died. But I recommend being very careful with this. It can't be changed even if the grantor has an argument with the beneficiary. For this reason, I personally prefer revocable trusts.

Another important benefit of trusts is that when a will is probated, it's part of the public record, while trusts are kept private.

So the main benefits of trusts, at least as they are set up in the United States, are that they allow the transfer of funds immediately upon death (revocable trust) or before death (irrevocable trust), save on court fees by bypassing probate, and are kept private from the public record.

This may make it sound like you don't need a will at all if you have a trust, but that is not the case. Let's talk about what's called a "pour-over will."

POUR-OVER WILL

A pour-over will is a last will and testament that serves as a "safety net" to catch any assets that were not included in a living trust.

All assets may not make it into a trust for a variety of reasons, so a pour-over will makes sure that all of the testator's property has been accounted for. Let's say the testator forgot to include their mother's antiques in the trust, or the testator might have bought property since the last time they updated their trust—those could be covered by a pour-over will. If you don't have a pour-over will, those assets would be handled as if you had died intestate.

Instead of a pour-over will, you can include the phrase "the rest and remainder of the estate" in your will, and anything not mentioned in the trust would then go to the beneficiary you designate in the will.

POWER OF ATTORNEY

A power of attorney document can designate someone to voice and execute many kinds of decisions, such as financial ones, that were previously set forth by the patient if they are unable to do it themselves. It is different from the health care proxy we discussed in chapter 2, which can only voice the patient's previously set forth medical decisions if they can't speak for themselves. The person who has been granted power of attorney works as the person's agent or attorney-in-fact. For this reason, your loved one may opt to have both of these documents in place. Just as the health care proxy must be carefully chosen, the person named in the power of attorney must also be chosen based on their trustworthiness and willingness to adhere to the patient's wishes. It also needs to be someone who can carry out the necessary tasks while perhaps in the midst of grief and strife.

Sometimes, people get executor and power of attorney mixed up as well. But an executor takes care of an estate *after* someone dies, while power of attorney is granted to someone while the patient is still alive. Once the person dies, the power of attorney ceases, and the executor takes over.

ADDING LOVED ONES' NAMES TO ACCOUNTS

When someone is close to end of life, it's a good idea for them to add the names of trusted loved ones to their bank accounts, safety deposit boxes, retirement accounts, and property titles. This makes it much easier for heirs to access the accounts and property without the usual stress and aggravation of probate, although the immediate permissions granted to them after the person's death will vary by state and country.

FINANCIAL PEACE OF MIND PLANNER CHECKLIST

Where's the title to Grandpa's Cadillac? Where are the keys to Mom's safe-deposit box? These are the kinds of things that can make our grief even more overwhelming than it already is. There's just no question that being organized helps everyone! Don't find yourself in the situation that Carla and her daughter experienced after Dan's death, as discussed earlier in this chapter.

Here's another cautionary tale for you: When Eleanor was diagnosed with stage 4 inoperable pancreatic cancer with only a few months to live, she finally created a will from her hospital bed, naming one friend, Donald, as her executor and another friend, Melissa, as her alternate executor. In her will, Eleanor bequeathed certain treasured items to friends and family members, and Donald took possession of them after Eleanor's death to hold until probate was completed. Then and only then would he be allowed to distribute the items to the beneficiaries named in Eleanor's will.

Sadly, nine months after Eleanor died, Donald died suddenly, leaving Melissa as the executor of Eleanor's estate. Except Donald didn't tell anyone where he had stored Eleanor's items to be distributed to her beneficiaries, and his widow was never able to locate them. As a result, none of Eleanor's friends and family received the items she wanted them to have. This is what happens when we don't tell someone else where important items are kept, and even an attorney can make this mistake.

As you can see, it's vital to keep a list of important items and passwords. Keep them in one place, and make sure to let at least two trusted people know where to find the information.

I know a woman who, along with her husband, met with a financial advisor to talk about their final plans. He asked her if she felt comfortable with the plan. She said, "Yes and no, because while I know I have all of the account numbers and passwords, I'm still not confident I could find them easily." As a result, they came up with the idea of a "financial fire drill." In that case, she had to collect the papers and make the calls as if her husband were dead. Every few months, they redo the drill to make sure all passwords and account numbers are current and that she can quickly locate everything.

Don't forget any of these items:

- ☐ Wills
- ☐ Trusts
- ☐ Advance directives
- ☐ Land deeds

- ☐ Mortgages
- ☐ Car and boat titles
- ☐ Powers of attorney
- ☐ Social Security card
- ☐ Safe-deposit box keys
- ☐ Veteran's benefits
- ☐ Passwords for all online accounts, including social media
- ☐ Stocks and bonds
- ☐ Where jewelry, heirlooms, and other property bequeathed in the will can be found
- ☐ Life insurance policies
- ☐ Retirement account information, including IRAs, 401Ks, etc.
- ☐ Bank account information
- ☐ Keys to property
- ☐ Mobile phone password
- ☐ Credit card account information
- ☐ Birth certificate

Lastly, does your loved one want to establish a scholarship or create an endowment of some kind before they die? If so, it's best to hire an attorney to facilitate these types of gifts.

The value of financial planning for peace of mind at the end of life is *priceless*, and I hope this chapter has shown you the importance of not putting it off. I also hope I've convinced you that it doesn't have to be as costly as you might have thought. Think of the great night's sleep you and your family will have once these matters have been addressed.

12

A Spiritual Good Death

> For those who seek to understand it, death is
> a highly creative force. The highest spiritual
> values of life can originate from the thought
> and study of death.
>
> —Dr. Elisabeth Kübler-Ross

I was in the middle of three consecutive twelve-hour shifts in the oncology unit—the kind that are actually fifteen or sixteen hours once you have completed your patients' charts and everything else. One of my patients was Madeline, a forty-four-year-old woman with gallbladder cancer, who came into the oncology unit on a Friday with a broken hip.

She was accompanied by her sister, Leslie, and both were in shock, completely blindsided that someone as young as Madeline could possibly break a hip. Her oncologist had failed to mention that chemotherapy can make a person's bones brittle.

In an effort to reduce their fears, I worked to build trust with the two women. Then we could concentrate on the broken hip and Madeline's ongoing cancer treatment.

By Saturday, her pain was under control, and the shock had

settled down. At about 6 p.m., I helped her use a bedside commode (a portable toilet for people who can't walk well). As I moved her back to bed—a one-step turn and pivot—she was suddenly out of breath. This was a completely new experience for her, as she'd had no prior lung or breathing issues. I asked her to sit still and breathe slowly. "Do you want the oxygen nasal cannula [a tube that provides oxygen through the nose]?" I asked. But Madeline shook her head no.

The room was quiet as I stood there with my hand on her shoulder. But both of us could feel that something serious was going on.

On Sunday morning, the night nurse told me that Madeline had continued to experience shortness of breath throughout the night. They ran several tests and determined that a blood clot from the hip fracture had traveled to her lung. Madeline continued to struggle to breathe all day, and her skin began to look pale, which indicated a decrease in blood circulation throughout her body.

On the weekends in our hospital, doctors did rounds whenever it worked for their schedule, and I had a habit of doing rounds with them so that I could hear what they said to and about my patients, as well as what the patient and family said to the doctors. In this way, I could make sure everyone clearly understood what the doctor told them, and I was in a better position to answer the questions that inevitably came up after the doctor left.

I arrived with Madeline's doctor for her rounds at 3:30 p.m., and as we crossed through the doorway, she said to the doctor, "I just want to thank you for everything you've done for me." When I turned to look at the doctor, tears were running down her face. Madeline was telling us she was going to die before any of us called it. How did she know this?

That night, at 10:39 p.m., she awoke from a nap and said, "Get my sister! I'm transitioning!" She said it with the excitement you'd hear from an eight-year-old child going to Disney World. The nurse quickly went to the family lounge to get her sister.

What did Madeline see? What did she know that not only removed her fear of dying, but left her exhilarated for her next chapter? We may never know (until we get there ourselves), but it's the kind of thing that often happens to people as they get close to death.

I have worked at the bedside of more than one thousand people at the end of life, and while they may not all declare, "I'm transitioning," I have seen countless numbers of them have similar experiences to Madeline's. It's a sacred, profound, and healing moment that I describe as the person getting their "spiritual eyes."

We saw this with Allie's father in the emotional good death chapter. He got his spiritual eyes, which allowed him to let go, forgive, and make sense of his life from a wiser point of view. This phenomenon is characterized by a complete shift in perspective when someone suddenly makes sense of all the puzzle pieces of their life and lets go of their fear of death. Everything begins to fit together, and they can reflect on all of their experiences with newfound clarity, understanding, and healing. They experience a deep sense of peace that not only benefits them but is a gift to their loved ones as well. It is, no question, a spiritual experience for them.

Spirituality is a term that's often thrown around but remains undefined for many people. Some associate it with a specific religion, while others see it as a quest for something higher and deeper in life. Put simply, I define spirituality as the connection we have with the world around us, transcending the physical realm into a deeper sense of self and meaning. Even for those who don't believe in an afterlife or a deity, it's interesting to see them be open to the possibility of spiritual experiences. Like the dying atheist who, when experiencing psychedelics, said she could only describe what felt like God's love, many people find a spiritual connection toward the end that they never anticipated and that brings them considerable peace.

WHAT IS SPIRITUAL PEACE OF MIND, AND WHY IS IT IMPORTANT?

Even though we can't know what happens after we die until we get there, it's amazing how people from all different backgrounds and religions say similar things as they get closer to leaving this world. No matter their background, whether strictly religious or atheist, they all share the same wisdom:

1. Everything happens for a reason, and the reason is to learn.
2. There is no judgment.
3. We are all connected to one universal consciousness. This consciousness is an Unconditional Force of Love also known as God, Higher Consciousness, Prana, Chi, the Tao, or other terms, depending on where you live and/or your culture/religious influences.

My personal belief (from all that I have seen) is that at the end of life, as our physical body begins to diminish, our spiritual body grows. As this continues, whether we lived in New York City or the far reaches of Siberia, we eventually receive spiritual wisdom that helps us make sense of everything that went on in our life.

Whatever you personally believe, spiritual peace of mind goes beyond the boundaries of religion or belief systems. It's a deeply personal journey that encompasses the realm of emotions, thoughts, and self-discovery. It's about looking within to *find a deeper sense of purpose and meaning, as we develop a connection with something greater than ourselves.*

A crucial aspect of spiritual peace of mind is understanding the interconnectedness of life. The concept of interconnectedness acknowledges that *we are all part of something greater,* and that *all living beings are linked and interdependent.* This connection helps us find compassion and empathy toward others, and it reinforces the importance of mindfulness and presence in our interactions.

Another element of spirituality is the ability to embrace the mystery of life—that there is more than meets the eye. It encourages us to explore the unknown and unexplainable, looking beyond the limitations of our senses to embrace the beauty and wonder of the world.

Spirituality encourages us to take responsibility for our actions. It emphasizes the importance of personal growth and development, and helps us reflect on our behaviors and beliefs, making changes where necessary. It inspires us to take action toward the betterment of ourselves and the world.

Finally, spirituality can help us find inner serenity and calm both in life and at the end of life. It reminds us that we are not defined by outward appearances or material possessions, but by our inner selves. It allows us to let go of worry and stress, focusing instead on the present moment.

THE "SOUL" ACROSS RELIGIONS AND CULTURES

Every major religion, in its own unique way, speaks about a non-physical, loving aspect of our being. This is frequently referred to as the soul, spirit, or inner self. It's seen as an integral part of us that transcends our physical existence and embodies love, compassion, and empathy. Here's a brief look at how various religions express this concept:

- **Christianity:** In Christianity, the soul is a nonphysical entity that is inherently good and capable of love. It's believed that every person has a soul that can connect with God through love and compassion.
- **Islam:** In Islam, the soul (Ruh) is a divine spark within us. It's seen as a source of love, kindness, and spiritual growth.
- **Hinduism:** The Atman, or soul, in Hinduism is eternal and inherently full of love. It's believed to be a fragment of the divine and seeks to reunite with the divine through love and compassion.
- **Buddhism:** While Buddhism does not directly speak of a soul, it refers to a concept known as Bodhicitta, the awakened heart that is full of compassion and love for all beings.
- **Judaism:** Judaism teaches the Neshama, a divine soul that is capable of unconditional love and kindness.
- **Sikhism:** Sikhism teaches about the "inner self" that is pure, loving, and eternally connected to God.

These teachings, although expressed differently, all point toward a nonphysical, loving aspect of us that transcends the physical world. By learning about and embracing this aspect, we can better understand ourselves and others, fostering compassion, empathy, and love in our lives.

Similarly, virtually every culture recognizes a nonphysical, loving aspect of our being, referred to by different names such as the soul, spirit, or inner self. Here's a brief look at how various cultures express this concept:

- **Native American cultures:** These cultures tend to believe in the existence of a spiritual self that is deeply connected to nature and other beings, as well as a source of love and compassion.
- **Indigenous Australian cultures:** Aboriginal culture believes in the Dreamtime, which is a spiritual concept that speaks of the soul's journey, emphasizing love, respect, and connection with all living beings.
- **African cultures:** Some African cultures believe in the concept of Ubuntu, which translates to "I am because we are" and represents a deep-rooted sense of compassion and respect for others, reflecting the nonphysical, loving part of us.
- **Eastern cultures:** Traditional cultures in India and China have referred to the concept of Atman or Chi, representing the nonphysical essence that is inherently loving and compassionate.
- **Western cultures:** While Western cultures may not explicitly talk about a nonphysical, loving component,

concepts like altruism, empathy, and love are deeply embedded in their societal values and moral philosophy.

All cultures seem to speak about a nonphysical part of us that transcends the physical body—after all, we are all united by death, regardless of culture, religion, or beliefs. This awareness can provide an enormous amount of comfort and peace when caring for someone at the end of life.

Is it simply that we just forgot? That the removal of death in our modern world has erased these ancient teachings that have been around for thousands of years and allow us to have a relationship with death that is based on global oneness, not fear?

THE BURDEN OF PROOF

It's true that no one can prove that a nonphysical part of us transcends the physical body when we die, but we can't disprove it either. I always feel that if you can't disprove something, why not choose to believe whatever brings the most peace and comfort now? Why not say *What if?* Why not stay open to the possibility that what the masses of people at end of life say is true?

What if there truly is no judgment? What if we are all connected? What if this life is all about learning unconditional love, and what if we *are* destined to see our deceased loved ones again? In my experience, that perspective alone brings a spiritual good death.

Seeking spiritual peace of mind encourages us to look beyond the physical world and to connect with something greater, helping us find purpose in life now and deeper meaning at the end of life. It teaches us the importance of compassion and empathy, as well as how we are all truly connected and so much more similar than we are different. By embracing spirituality, we can find inner peace, calm, fulfillment, compassion, empathy, and connection. It's an invitation to embrace the mysteries, wonders, and beauty of life, death, and the world.

SPIRITUAL PEACE OF MIND PLANNER

What can you do to enhance your spiritual peace of mind whether you are at end of life or helping someone else prepare for theirs? Here are some strategies I recommend:

1. **Meditation:** Regular meditation can calm the mind, reduce stress, and promote inner peace. It's a practice embraced by many cultures and religions worldwide.
2. **Mindfulness:** Being present in each moment can help you appreciate life's simple pleasures and reduce anxiety about the past or future.
3. **Prayer or spiritual reflection:** Many find solace and peace in prayer or reflecting on spiritual teachings, regardless of their religious affiliation.
4. **Nature walks:** Spending time in nature can foster a deep connection with the world around you, promoting a sense of peace and tranquility.
5. **Gratitude practice:** Regularly expressing gratitude can shift your focus from what's wrong to what's right in your life, which people report leads to greater contentment and peace.

6. **Community connection:** Participating in community activities can nourish your sense of belonging, enhancing spiritual peace.

7. **Personal growth:** Pursuing personal growth through learning, self-reflection, and embracing new experiences can contribute to spiritual peace of mind.

THE FASTEST WAY TO SPIRITUAL CONNECTION: SERVICE

Everyone is searching for fulfillment. We are told we can achieve this by working hard, going to college, getting a "good job," marrying the "perfect spouse," buying a big house with a fence, and having two or more children. But what I have learned from the wisdom of those in the last weeks of life is that these things are *not* it. From what they have said, true fulfillment can only come from an energetic alignment with a higher connection to something greater than us, and that higher connection can only be achieved by being of service to others in some way without a sense of obligation or an attachment to the outcome. It's the absolute fastest way I know to connect to spiritual energy. The best experiences of my life have been the things I have done from a place of pure giving without the need for the recipients to reciprocate. This can incorporate simply smiling at someone, holding the door open for them, lending an ear to someone who is upset, or going so far as to do volunteer work.

Certainly, if you're caring for your loved one at end of life, you are doing a great service. And, of course, as we've already covered, it's important to also take care of yourself during any time of service and make sure you don't overspend your personal resources. Nevertheless, the secret that service is the root of true happiness and spiritual connection has been known by some of the greatest minds in this world for all of time:

> "WE MAKE A LIVING BY WHAT WE GET, BUT WE MAKE
> A LIFE BY WHAT WE GIVE."
> —*Winston Churchill*

> "ONLY A LIFE LIVED FOR OTHERS IS A LIFE
> WORTHWHILE."
> —*Albert Einstein*

> "I DON'T KNOW WHAT YOUR DESTINY WILL BE, BUT
> ONE THING I DO KNOW: THE ONLY ONES AMONG YOU
> WHO WILL BE REALLY HAPPY ARE THOSE WHO HAVE
> SOUGHT AND FOUND HOW TO SERVE."
> —*Albert Schweitzer*

> "WE ARE NOT PUT ON THIS EARTH FOR OURSELVES,
> BUT ARE PLACED HERE FOR EACH OTHER. IF YOU ARE
> THERE ALWAYS FOR OTHERS, THEN IN TIME OF NEED,
> SOMEONE WILL BE THERE FOR YOU."
> —*Jeff Warner*

> "HE WHO WISHES TO SECURE THE GOOD OF OTHERS
> HAS ALREADY SECURED HIS OWN."
> —*Confucius*

"THE BEST WAY TO FIND YOURSELF IS TO LOSE YOUR-
SELF IN THE SERVICE OF OTHERS."
—*Mahatma Gandhi*

"NEVER DOUBT THAT A SMALL GROUP OF THOUGHT-
FUL, COMMITTED CITIZENS CAN CHANGE THE WORLD;
INDEED, IT'S THE ONLY THING THAT EVER HAS."
—*Margaret Mead*

"EVERYONE CAN BE GREAT, BECAUSE EVERYONE CAN
SERVE."
—*Martin Luther King Jr.*

"I HAVE FOUND THAT AMONG ITS OTHER BENEFITS,
GIVING LIBERATES THE SOUL OF THE GIVER."
—*Maya Angelou*

Epilogue

DEATH AS A SACRED EXPERIENCE

> Death opens us up to the true reality of our
> inner being and selfhood.
>
> —Victor Frankl

Death used to be seen as a sacred rite of passage. In many cultures throughout history, it was viewed as a ceremonial event marking the transition from one spiritual form to another. It was honored and revered as an important phase of life.

Today, unfortunately, we have lost this sacred connection to death, which can be our greatest teacher about life. It teaches us the difference between the two main guiding forces within us all: ego-based guidance and heart-centered guidance. Ego-based guidance leads us to make decisions out of fear and selfishness, while heart-centered guidance leads us to make decisions from a place of love of self, others, and all of life.

When we hold space for someone at the end of their life and are privileged to witness a good death, we're granted access to the heart-centered guidance system that can bestow life-changing wisdom on us. We're allowed to bear witness to the dissolution of that person's ego (the human part of them) and the subsequent emergence of their soul self before they leave this world. We can never look at life the same way after being part of this experience. Saying goodbye (for now) to those we love will never be easy, but when we know the true sacredness that surrounds this beautiful transition, we are never the same.

The minute I started working with the dying, my entire life changed. I noticed right away that as they neared the end, the majority of people reached a place of spiritual peace. So many of them said the same things, regardless of their religion or culture, or even if they were atheists. It was as though they had solved a puzzle. It was clear to me that everything was not only going to be all right, but it was divinely orchestrated the entire time. They had received their "spiritual eyes."

THREE DIFFERENT PHENOMENA AT THE END OF LIFE

In 2023 hospice nurse Hadley Vlahos wrote a book called *The In Between: Unforgettable Encounters During Life's Final Moments*, which shares stories from her dying patients. It soared to the top of the *New York Times* bestseller list and stayed there for fourteen weeks. Obviously, people are hungry for this information and the comfort it provides. What she wrote aligns with my experience as a hospice nurse and death doula.

There are three different phenomena that I have experienced countless times with patients at the end of life. Again, it happens universally regardless of a person's religion, culture, or background.

1. People get a surge of energy.

When I was a relatively new hospice nurse, I had a new patient named Patricia who was eighty-three years old. She was a tall woman with thick silver hair that came to her shoulders. Sadly, she fell in her bathroom and was not found for two days. By that time, she was close to death. Her family was distraught and confused how it could have happened. As I tended to her, I tried to connect with her, but Patricia could hardly hold her head up or utter an audible word.

The next day, I walked in and saw her grandson, who was twenty-five, sitting in the sunroom where Patricia's hospital bed had been placed. As I walked through the door facing him, I heard a woman say, "Hello!" I turned around and saw Patricia looking right at me, clear as a bell. Then she asked, "Who are you?"

I said, "I'm the nurse, and I'm here to see how you're doing."

Her grandson saw the surprised expression on my face and said, "I know! She's been like this since last night." He said she woke up and asked for Baileys Irish Cream and pizza.

"What did you do?" I asked.

"I gave them to her."

"Good!" I answered.

I had no idea what was going on, but I asked a seasoned hospice nurse about it. She said, "Oh, yeah, that's the surge of energy. It often happens right before a person dies. They 'wake up' and can be clearer than they've been in twenty or thirty years."

My friend Melanie tells the story of her beloved friend Keith, who was dying of AIDS at age twenty-nine back in the 1990s before the medications we have today. She says he was the funniest person she ever met. He could tell stories at a party and have everyone there doubled over with laughter.

Soon after he entered the hospital, he was in a sleep coma for days. But as people gathered around his bed to say goodbye to him, he suddenly awakened and gave a final performance with as much energy as he ever had. He had everyone in stitches and then went back into his sleep coma, dying shortly thereafter.

This surge of energy, often referred to as the "end of life rally," is a fascinating phenomenon that occurs in the final days or hours of a person's life. It's a period when they suddenly "wake up" with an unexpected burst of energy, mental clarity, and/or physical function. This happens to people despite their weakened state due to illness or aging.

The surge can last from an hour to several days. I usually see it for a twelve-hour period. It provides a special opportunity for loved ones to say anything they still want and need to say. It's a moment for final goodbyes and expressions of love. You can't get more sacred than that.

Of course, this doesn't occur with everyone, and it's important to understand that it *is not a sign of recovery*, but rather a gift at the end of life.

2. People can control the time they die.

People nearing the end of their lives seem to have some control over the timing of their death. They may hold on until a significant date, an important event, or the arrival or departure of a loved one. Often, they wait for what *they* consider the "right" time to die, which may or may not coincide with what we, as their loved ones, consider the right time.

There are four main reasons why someone will wait to die:

1. **Waiting for someone to come to their bedside.**
2. **Waiting for someone to leave the room.** Conversely, people often wait for us to leave their bedside before they will go. This happens so often, in fact, that we even instruct families to leave the room for a period of time if their loved one is lingering beyond the expected one to three days in an active dying coma. Maybe they're trying to protect us from witnessing the moment of their transition, or perhaps they don't want their death to be our last memory of them. One of my students casually mentioned this truth to an eighty-three-year-old man, who began to cry when he was told that people often wait until we leave before they take their last breath. "You just gave me the greatest gift I could ever ask for," he told her. "I have been holding on to guilt for thirty-five years that I wasn't with my mother when she died. Thank you so much." How does someone in a sleeping coma for days know that we have just left the room? Well, we know that hearing is the last of the senses to go. So it's very likely that the dying person can hear what's going on in the room even after they can no longer respond. For this reason, always talk softly, and be mindful of what you say in their presence. Waiting for us to leave is believed to be a final act of love on the part of the dying, as they spare us from seeing their death and allow us to maintain our happiest memories from our lives together.
3. **Waiting for permission to go.** Often, it helps if family or friends give the dying person permission to go.

They might be worried about the people they're leaving behind. So you can say something like, "If you need to go, I understand. I love you, and I'll miss you. But I'll be okay. I don't want you to suffer anymore. It's okay to go." I have seen many, many people die peacefully within minutes of receiving this permission.

4. **Waiting for a significant date or matter to be resolved.** Some people appear to delay their death until a particular moment that holds significance for them, such as a birthday, anniversary, or the arrival of a baby in the family.

The story of Aunt Bessie is an example of the fourth reason. She was ninety-nine years old and a little bird of a thing. She had one daughter, Gail, who was her sole caregiver and aged seventy-three herself. On my first visit with Aunt Bessie, she could not have been more wonderful. She was smiling and in no pain, and she had the cutest feet I have ever seen.

That night, Aunt Bessie went into her deep sleep coma. But day three came, then day four, and she lingered on. Science tells us the human body can't live without water for longer than three days, but the days of Aunt Bessie's sleeping coma extended to ten, all without water. What was happening?

Every day, I went to the house to check on her and to support Gail. I asked her the typical questions, such as "Is she waiting for someone to come?" But Gail insisted the answer was no.

"We all thought she was going to die last summer," Gail told me, "so we had a huge family reunion. Everyone was there."

The next question I asked was "Are you giving her alone time?"

Gail assured me that she was. In fact, she was sleeping in another room.

Baffled and confused, I went back to the hospice office to work on my patients' charts. It was there I noticed that Aunt Bessie's one hundredth birthday was just five days away. "She's waiting to turn one hundred!" I thought to myself. And that's exactly what she did. Aunt Bessie turned one hundred and had a peaceful transition into the next world at 4:04 a.m.

3. People will talk about being visited by loved ones who have already died.

One of the most intriguing, inspiring, and healing phenomena during end-of-life stages is that individuals frequently report seeing and speaking to loved ones who have already passed away. These experiences are often vivid, and they can be comforting and reassuring for those nearing the end of their lives.

According to studies, up to 72 percent of dying individuals report these experiences, which usually occur when they are awake, not just in dreams. While some people may dismiss these as hallucinations or the effects of medication, many health care professionals and researchers consider them a significant part of the dying process. Understanding this phenomenon, which offers the possibility that we go on, can help families and caregivers heal from grief and know that their dying loved one will be okay. It's important for family members to listen to the dying person, validate these experiences, and understand that this is a sign they will be physically leaving the world soon.

My patient Helen, who was in her early nineties, experienced this phenomenon. Aside from a few chronic illnesses, she was simply in hospice care for being old. We call this hospice diagnosis "failure to thrive." But to meet hospice criteria, we need to show that a person is steadily decreasing in health by a measurable outcome. If we can't show this (usually by weight loss) with the diagnosis of "failure to thrive," the patient "graduates" and is "kicked off" hospice care. Helen would come on hospice services and get kicked off twelve weeks later. Six months would go by, and she'd be admitted again. This went on for two years. We all got to know her and her family very well, and we loved them all.

One Sunday, I was at a local farmers' market and ran into Helen's daughter, Debbie. We were excited to see each other, and with a big smile, Debbie said, "Did you ever hear how my mom died?" I hadn't. She said that her family took turns caring for Helen in her final days. One day while her adult niece, Jill, was watching over her, Helen suddenly said, "Bob was here last night. He looked so handsome. And he said he's coming Saturday to take me to the dance!" Bob was Helen's husband who had died twenty years earlier. With some anxiety in her voice, Helen said, "I need something to wear!"

Jill went upstairs and retrieved one of Helen's best Sunday dresses. "How is this?" she asked Helen.

"Perfect!" Helen said. Jill hung the dress on the back of the bedroom door where Helen could see it.

The next day, Helen exclaimed, "Shoes! I need shoes for the dance!" Jill brought down a pair of red patent leather shoes that Helen always loved and put them on the floor next to the dress.

When Saturday came, Helen died in her sleep in a complete state of peace. I like to think of her dancing with Bob in her beautiful dress and red shoes.

THE COMMON THINGS DYING PEOPLE SAY

As people get closer to the time of death, they frequently say the same things—again, regardless of their religion, culture, or beliefs. Here are the four main things they commonly share with the living before they die:

1. There is *no* death.
2. Everything happens for a reason.
3. There is no judgment.
4. We are all connected to one unconditionally loving energy.

These are the same words of wisdom that are expressed in studies of near-death experiences and by people who use psychedelics to reduce fear at the end of life. There is something to this, and it's life-changing information.

A GOOD DEATH IS A GOOD LIFE, BUT WHAT DOES THAT MEAN?

Death may be a sacred experience, but *so is this life*. The most peaceful end-of-life experiences I have been privileged and honored to witness were from those who had lived a full life—not in the sense of material things, but in love, presence, and appreciation. From those experiences, this is my best advice:

- Follow your heart to align with your purpose.
- Treat each day like one little lifetime.
- Know that time is your greatest commodity. How you choose

> to spend it and who you choose to spend it with are the most
> important decisions you will make.

WAYS YOU CAN FACILITATE A SACRED
EXPERIENCE FOR YOUR LOVED ONE

If you feel it's appropriate, you can share the information in this
chapter with your loved one. Many times at the end of life, people
are more open than they might have been in the past, as they seek
a greater knowing. They are looking for that glimmer of possibility
that there is more, and just that one little possibility may be all it
takes to give them a more beautiful end-of-life experience.

Sometimes, you don't need to say anything at all, of course. You can
take cues from one another. If *you* are not afraid and are grounded in
your belief that there's more, they will feel that too. I know as a hospice
nurse working with the dying for years, when I went into a home and
was as grounded, present, and loving as possible, the energy of everyone
there also shifted. I believe they thought, "Well, if she's not freaking out,
and she does this all the time, maybe we don't have to freak out either."

Just consider these questions:

- What if we have death all wrong?
- What if death is just a "graduation" to another world?
- What if the present way we live, with the removal of
  death awareness and education, is creating chaos, sep-
  arateness, and fear?
- Could death be the greatest teacher about how to live,
  not just for ourselves, but for the entire world?

My intention in writing this book has been to empower you with the skills to care for someone you love at the end of life so that it can be the most positive experience possible. I want to help you soften your grief and give you the hope that you will see your loved one again and that they will always be with you.

I believe wholeheartedly that there is so much more going on in this life than most of us are aware of. That *more* is the beingness of all things and our connection to unconditional love. It's a miraculous place to know and live within, and it's accessible to all of us at any time. We just have to surrender to it.

May your loved one have a good death, and may you also have a good death when your time comes.

"FOR WHAT IS IT TO DIE BUT TO STAND NAKED IN THE
WIND AND TO MELT INTO THE SUN?...
AND WHEN THE EARTH SHALL CLAIM YOUR LIMBS,
THEN SHALL YOU TRULY DANCE."
—*Kahlil Gibran*

Acknowledgments

First, I would like to thank Kris Carr. You put me on the path of clarity and acceleration. Your mentorship, guidance, and laughter are priceless.

To Richelle Fredson, thank you for keeping on me and reminding me that I needed to write this book when I could not even wrap my head around how I would do that with my Doulagivers teaching schedule. You made the proposal process not only seamless, but quick and fun. You are the absolute expert in your field.

To my literary agents, Jan Baumer and Steve Troha, thank you for trusting me enough to push me out of my comfort zone and challenging me to make the best prescriptive end-of-life educational book I could possibly make. The results are amazing!

To Marisa Vigilante, thank you for seeing this vision and launching this project.

To Thea Diklich-Newell, thank you for all your edits and incredible feedback. I am deeply moved.

To my editor, Cara Bedick, thank you for adding insightful feedback to this book and encouraging me to add a chapter that significantly shaped this manuscript.

To my publisher, Michael Szczerban, and the entire team at Little, Brown Spark, thank you for believing in my vision and bringing this book to life. I could not ask for a better group of talented and vision-focused people to do this with.

To Melanie Votaw, your ability to bring words to the page with clarity and warmth are unmatched. You are so gifted. I will always be grateful to have had you by my side during this journey. You are not only a brilliant writer, but an incredible human being.

Thank you to all the death doulas who are stepping forward, following their calling, and changing the end of life to once again be the natural, sacred experience it was meant to be.

To my family, thank you for all the love and support throughout the years. What a miraculous journey.

To my son, Nicholas, the love you saw in me allowed me to (over time) see it in myself. We would not be here without you. May I be that light for others on their journey.

Finally, but most importantly, I express my deepest thanks to all the patients and families who have allowed me to be part of your journeys. You have not only taught me everything about the end of life, but have taught me everything about *life*. You each have a place in my heart.

Thank you all for being a part of this journey. I hope this book brings you empowerment, peace, and inspiration to have not only a good death, but a good life.

xo Suzanne

Glossary

ADVANCE DIRECTIVES: documents that allow us to plan and make our own end-of-life wishes known in the event that we are unable to communicate. Advance directives consist of a living will and a health care proxy document.

BENEFICIARY: someone named in a last will and testament, trust, or life insurance policy who is to receive money or property from the person creating the document.

BEQUEST: a gift given to a beneficiary in a last will and testament, which can be money or most anything else. When a bequest is given to someone, it is "bequeathed" to them.

CPR: cardiopulmonary resuscitation to attempt to get someone's heart started after it has stopped.

DNR: Do Not Resuscitate order to prevent medical personnel from performing CPR.

EXECUTOR: the person named in a last will and testament who files the will with the probate court, sees to it that the testator's wishes are fulfilled, and distributes possessions to the beneficiaries named in the will.

FEEDING TUBE: a medical device used to provide nutrition to people who cannot obtain nutrition by mouth, are unable to swallow safely, or need nutritional supplementation.

FIVE STAGES OF GRIEF: developed by Dr. Elisabeth Kübler-Ross, the five stages (in no particular order) are denial, anger, bargaining, depression, and acceptance.

GRANNY POD: a small, detached guest house with a bedroom, bathroom, living area, and kitchenette that can be placed in a backyard (also called an accessory dwelling unit or ADU).

GRANTOR: a person who has funds or property they want to give to someone else at a particular time via a trust (also sometimes called a trustor).

HEALTH CARE PROXY (HCP): a health care proxy document allows us to appoint someone we trust, such as a family member or close friend, to voice our health care decisions if we lose the ability to speak for ourselves. By appointing a health care proxy, we can make sure that health care providers follow our wishes. A health care proxy may also be called a health care surrogate, health care power of attorney, medical power of attorney, or health care agent.

HOSPICE: a special kind of care that strives to maintain a person's dignity and quality of life, including pain control, as they near end of life.

IRREVOCABLE TRUST: a trust that cannot be changed once it has been signed.

LAST WILL AND TESTAMENT: a legal document in which we express our wishes as to how our possessions are to be distributed after our death, whether it's money, property, or personal items. We may also specify our wishes in this document about our funeral or service, what should happen to our body after death, how our debts and taxes will be paid, and who might serve as guardians for our children or pets.

LIVING TRUST: a trust that is in effect while the grantor is still living.

LIVING WILL: an advance directive document detailing a person's desires regarding their medical treatment if they are no longer able to express informed consent.

MEDICAL AID IN DYING (MAID): a medical practice in which a terminally ill, mentally capable adult may request a prescription from their doctor for medication to end their life.

NOTARIZATION: the official process by which a notary public witnesses someone sign a document and verifies their identity by checking their identification. The notary public then signs the document as well and applies their official stamp to the document.

PALLIATIVE CARE: treatment that relieves symptoms but doesn't cure the illness. It's used to make people comfortable when their illness can't be cured.

PALLIATIVE SEDATION: a state induced by ongoing medication intended to keep a dying person asleep and comfortable (also sometimes called terminal sedation, continuous deep sedation, or sedation for intractable distress of a dying patient).

POLST/MOLST: a legally binding medical order that sets forth medical instructions in a standardized format to address key critical care decisions consistent with the patient's goals of care and clinical results. It is designed to facilitate shared, informed medical decision-making and communication between health care professionals and patients with advanced, progressive illness or frailty. It can only be created when someone has been given a serious illness diagnosis. POLST stands for physician orders for life-sustaining treatment, and MOLST stands for medical orders for life-sustaining treatment; they are just different names for the same thing.

POUR-OVER WILL: a last will and testament that serves as a safety device to capture any assets that have not been transferred to or included in a living trust.

POWER OF ATTORNEY (POA): a document that names someone as a person's agent or attorney-in-fact with specific powers that are set forth within the document.

PROBATE: the legal process that establishes the validity and authenticity of someone's last will and testament after they die. The court where probate is done reviews the assets of the estate and determines what estate taxes, if any, must be paid to the government.

PSILOCYBIN: a psychedelic chemical obtained from certain types of fresh or dried mushrooms. Psilocybin is being used in trials to treat acute fear of death. Dr. Anthony P. Bossis of the New York University School of Medicine states in his study that dying patients who took psilocybin described having feelings of wonder, awe, humility, gratitude, transcendence, and transformation. For the treatment of the acute fear of death, studies have found that just one standard dose is enough to recalibrate how someone feels about dying.

REVOCABLE TRUST: a trust that can be changed or dissolved by the grantor during their lifetime. A revocable trust becomes irrevocable once the grantor dies.

TESTATOR: the person who creates a last will and testament to distribute their possessions after their death.

TRUST: a financial arrangement that allows a trustee or third party to hold assets owned by a grantor for the benefit of a beneficiary or beneficiaries.

TRUSTEE: the person who is responsible for seeing that the beneficiaries of a trust receive the assets named in the trust at the time specified.

VOLUNTARILY STOPPING EATING AND DRINKING (VSED): a process, legal in all fifty US states, whereby the patient decides to stop eating at end of life, which usually causes death within seven to fourteen days and mimics the natural way the body dies.

Appendix A

Prolonged grief disorder occurs when someone is unable to engage in activities essential to daily quality of life six months or a year after a death or loss. While everyone grieves in their own time, and the pain of losing someone or something may never completely go away, the heaviness should lessen over time. When it doesn't, and it keeps us from activities of daily living like bathing, eating properly, and socializing, it may be a sign of prolonged grief disorder.

If this is happening to you or someone you know, it's important to reach out for therapeutic support. When it gets to this stage, it usually can't be healed without help, and there's certainly no shame in asking for help. A therapist trained in grief counseling will have specific strategies for moving beyond the grief and participating fully in life again.

Appendix B

WHAT TO SAY TO SOMEONE WHO'S GRIEVING

Even if you are the caregiver for someone who has died, you may feel you want to help someone else in your family or circle through their grieving process. You might be grieving at the same time, but it can still be difficult to know what to say.

First, remember that it's mostly about being with them in true presence. Just showing up in a loving, compassionate, and nonjudgmental way will help them immensely. Also, rather than talking, just try listening to them.

Understand that it isn't your job to "fix" them or try to cheer them up. Allow them to be with their feelings. Let them know that you will be with them as they walk this path. With that in mind, here are some things you can say:

> What can I do for you?
> I'm here for you.
> Please know how much I care.
> You can call me anytime.
> I'm holding you in my thoughts and prayers.
> Can you share some of your favorite stories about them with me?

Appendix C

1. Take your time.
2. Be present.
3. Lean into the grief, knowing that it's a natural and expected process. Honoring it will help you move through it.
4. Talk about it. Find a support group, if possible. Speaking about your grief with others who understand will help you heal.
5. Write in a Grief Journal about your feelings.
6. Reframe the experience with a "highlight reel" of your positive memories.
7. Practice self-forgiveness for anything you feel guilty about. Practice forgiveness of the person you lost with regard to any unresolved anger or blame.
8. Practice gratitude. In positive psychology research, gratitude is strongly and consistently associated with greater happiness. It helps people feel more positive emotions, relish good experiences, improve their health, deal with adversity, and build stronger relationships.[1]

9. Be of service. Scientific research provides compelling data to support giving as a powerful pathway to happiness. Through fMRI technology, we now know that giving activates the same parts of the brain that are stimulated by food and sex. So altruism is hardwired in the brain to be pleasurable.[2] Helping others may just be the secret to healing from grief and living a healthier, wealthier, more productive, and meaningful life.

10. Our Doulagivers Level 1 Training includes healing from grief. The following are comments by people who have participated in this training and found relief:

"I WAS DRAWN TO THIS SESSION IN A SEARCH FOR A MEANINGFUL AND EFFECTIVE GRIEF GUIDE.
I KNOW THIS SESSION WAS ACTUALLY FOCUSED ON DEATH DOULAS AND HELPING OTHERS THROUGH THE END-OF-LIFE PROCESS, BUT IT WAS ALSO THE MOST USEFUL TOOL I HAVE SEEN IN PROCESSING LOSS AND GRIEF. I HAD TRIED GRIEF COUNSELING WITH TWO THERAPISTS AND ATTENDED SEVERAL ONLINE GRIEF SUPPORT WORKSHOPS. I HAD YET TO FIND ANY OF THAT HELPFUL IN ANY WAY. I WAS FRUSTRATED IN NOT BEING ABLE TO RESOLVE MY OWN GRIEF, BUT EVEN MORE SO FOR THE OTHERS WHO WERE GRIEVING ALONGSIDE ME. . . . I WAS DISAPPOINTED IN NOT FINDING A HELPFUL RESOURCE.
THIS TRAINING HAS BEEN SO AMAZING, I CAN SEE HOW CLOSELY IT IS RELATED TO GRIEF AND PROCESSING LOSS. I WANT TO THANK YOU FOR THIS

FREE SESSION.... I APPRECIATE YOU; I WANT TO LEARN
MORE ABOUT BEING A DEATH DOULA AND
FOLLOW THIS JOURNEY DEEPER.
I FEEL VERY CONNECTED HERE."
—*Kristen*

"THANK YOU SO MUCH. WHEN MY SON DIED, I JUST
FELT BROKEN WHEN HE KEPT SAYING HE WANTED TO
GO HOME. I REPLIED THAT HE WAS HOME. I GET IT
NOW. HE WAS TELLING HIS MOMMA HE WANTED TO
GO AND THAT WAS HIS GOODBYE. THANK YOU."
—*Theresa*

"THANK YOU! THANK YOU! THANK YOU! I FEEL HEALED
FROM MY PARENTS' DEATH ISSUES THAT I HAVE
CARRIED FOR THE LAST FORTY-PLUS YEARS. I LEARNED
SO MUCH. YOUR COMPASSION COMES THROUGH EVERY
WORD. I CAN'T THANK YOU ENOUGH FOR SHARING
THIS BEAUTIFUL JOURNEY."
—*Viv*

Appendix D

HOW TO TALK TO KIDS ABOUT DEATH

I personally believe that much of our denial of the reality of death and our fear of death are the result of our parents trying to protect and shield us when we were children. We have set ourselves up in our society for a dysfunctional relationship with death.

I also believe that the best service we can offer children is to talk to them honestly about death. When we skirt the issue and deny the truth, it only causes them to feel more afraid. This communicates that something's wrong rather than a natural process.

Someone recently said, "If a child is old enough to ask a question, they're old enough to get an answer." I agree. Of course, what we say must be age-appropriate.

If a child is struggling to accept someone's death, please get them counseling if at all possible. Meanwhile, there are books available to help you with what to say, as well as organizations like the Dougy Center at Dougy.org.

Resources

Doulagivers

All free resources: https://doulagivers.com/free-resource-page

Family Caregiver Community on Facebook: https://www.facebook
.com/groups/doulagivers.family.caregiver.community

Level 1 End-of-Life Doula and Family Caregiver Training Webinar: https://doulagivers.com/monthly-free-class-register

Level 1 End-of-Life Doula Training—Veterans Edition: https://
www.doulagivers.com/doulagivers-level-one-veterans-edition

Death Doula Discovery Webinar: https://doulagivers.com
/practitioner-webinar

Life Cafe: https://doulagivers.zoom.us/meeting/register
/u5MrceChpz4otzcgvm6APV3KQkhdWpzBKg

Death Doula Guide: https://www.doulagivers.com/death-doula
-guide-2

Caregiver Checklist: https://doulagivers.com/caregiver-checklist

Forgiveness Guide: https://www.facebook.com/groups/doulagivers
.family.caregiver.community

Grief Guide: https://www.doulagivers.com/grief

9 Choice Advance Directive: https://www.doulagivers.com/the
-doulagivers-9-choice-advance-directive

CaringBridge (allows you to provide updates to loved ones about someone's condition): https://www.caringbridge.org

Dougy Center (for help with talking to kids about death): https://www.dougy.org

Notes

Chapter 1: We Become Less Fearful of the Unknown When We Embrace What Is Known

1   Aaron O'Neill. "Life Expectancy in the United States, 1860–2020. *Statista.* June 21, 2022. https://www.statista.com /statistics/1040079/life-expectancy-united-states-all-time.

2   Saloni Dattani, Lucas Rodés-Guirao, Hannah Ritchie, Esteban Ortiz-Ospina, and Max Roser. "Life Expectancy." *Our World in Data.* 2023. https://ourworldindata.org/life-expectancy.

3   World Health Organization. "Palliative Care." *World Health Organization Newsroom Fact Sheets.* August 5, 2020. https:// www.who.int/news-room/fact-sheets/detail/palliative-care.

4   Phyllis Shacter. "Not Here by Choice." *TEDx Bellingham.* November 25, 2013. https://www.phyllisshacter.com/transcript-of -expanded-tedx-presentation.

5   Paula Span. "The VSED Exit: A Way to Speed Up Dying, Without Asking Permission." *New York Times.* October 21, 2016. https://www.nytimes.com/2016/10/25/health /voluntarily-stopping-eating-drinking.html.

6   Tanya Lewis. "Johns Hopkins Scientists Give Psychedelics the Serious Treatment." *Scientific American.* January 16, 2020. https://www.scientificamerican.com/article/johns-hopkins -scientists-give-psychedelics-the-serious-treatment.

7   Anthony P. Bossis. "Psychedelics and Psychology: Modern Medicine Meets Ancient Medicine." *TEDx Talks YouTube.* October 18, 2017. https://www.youtube.com/watch?v =U561dQIe6c4.

Chapter 2:
Preparing for Longer Lifespans: The Elder Care Crisis

1   Nancy Oehieng, Juliette Cubanski, Tricia Neuman, and Anthony Damico. "How Many Older Adults Live in Poverty?" *KFF.* May 21, 2024. https://www.kff.org/medicare/issue-brief/how -many-older-adults-live-in-poverty.

2   Penn Medicine. "Two Out of Three U.S. Adults Have Not Completed an Advance Directive." *Penn Medicine News.* July 5, 2017. https://www.pennmedicine.org/news/news -releases/2017/july/two-out-of-three-us-adults-have-not -completed-an-advance-directive.

Chapter 6:
The Rebirth of Death

1   "The Case for Home Funerals." *Sacred Crossings.* Accessed October 1, 2023. https://sacredcrossings.com/the-case-for -home-funerals.

2   Rebecca Lake, Heidi Gollub, and Kara McGinley. "How Much Does a Funeral Cost in 2023?" *USA Today.* September 27, 2023. https://www.usatoday.com/money/blueprint/life-insurance /how-much-does-a-funeral-cost.

Chapter 7:
Keeping Death Green: How Our Funeral and Burial Choices Impact the Planet

1   United Nations. "World Social Report 2023: Leaving No One Behind in an Ageing World." *United Nations Department of Economic and Social Affairs.* Accessed May 3, 2024. https:// www.un.org/development/desa/dspd/wp-content/uploads /sites/22/2023/01/WSR_2023_Chapter_Key_Messages.pdf.

2   Allie Yang. "Rest in…Compost? These 'Green Funerals' Offer an Eco-Friendly Afterlife." February 24, 2023. https://www .nationalgeographic.com/environment/article/rest-in-compost -these-green-funerals-offer-an-eco-friendly-afterlife.

Chapter 10: An Emotional Good Death

1   Johns Hopkins Medicine. "Forgiveness: Your Health Depends on It." *Johns Hopkins Medicine.* Accessed January 5, 2024. https://www.hopkinsmedicine.org/health/wellness-and -prevention/forgiveness-your-health-depends-on-it.

Chapter 11: A Financial Good Death

1   Daniel de Visé. "Where's the Inheritance? Why Fewer Older Americans Are Writing Wills or Estate Planning." *USA Today.* October 4, 2023. https://www.usatoday.com/story/money /personalfinance/2023/10/03/fewer-older-americans-are -writing-wills-planning-estates/70994383007.

Appendix C: Your Loving Reminder Checklist to Heal from Grief

1   Harvard Medical School. "Giving Thanks Can Make You Happier." *Harvard Health Publishing.* August 14, 2021. https:// www.health.harvard.edu/healthbeat/giving-thanks-can-make -you-happier.

2   Vicki Contie. "Brain Imaging Reveals Joys of Giving." *National Institutes of Health.* June 22, 2007. https://www.nih.gov/news -events/nih-research-matters/brain-imaging-reveals-joys -giving.

Index

About the Author

SUZANNE B. O'BRIEN is a living, breathing example of what it's like to find your purpose. A former hospice and oncology nurse turned Doulagivers trainer, she has dedicated her life to teaching people how to care for those at the end of it. Considered a pioneer in the global Death Doula movement, Suzanne is a sought-after and respected teacher who has taught Doulagivers Training to people all around the world, including Buddhist monks who specialize in end-of-life care in Thailand.

Her work has been featured in major media outlets, including the *New York Times, Oprah Magazine, Hospice Times,* CBS News, and more. She was featured in the *Time* magazine article "Death Doulas Used to Be Rare. The Covid-19 Pandemic Changed That." In 2019, she was also named Humanitarian Ambassador for *Oprah Magazine* (now *Oprah Daily*).

Suzanne's Doulagivers Institute provides free education on how to care for someone who is dying through her Level 1 End-of-Life Doula Training program. Every month, this training is offered live online and gets between 2,500 and 5,000 registrations from every part of the world. To date, she has given this training to more than 360,000 people in more than 34 countries.

Suzanne recently launched the "How to Care for Someone Who Is Dying: The Good Death" Doulagivers Global Initiative (DGI).

This is part of a global campaign to bring death back to being the natural, sacred experience it once was by offering the free Level 1 Doulagivers Training to empower, heal, and inspire more people.

Awarded "Worldwide Leader in Health Care" by the International Nurses Association, Suzanne is the former vice president and founding member of the National End-of-Life Doula Alliance, a founding member of the End-of-Life Doula Council from the National Hospice and Palliative Care Organization, and the founder and creator of World Training Day, the Annual Death Doula Global Summit, and National Death Doula Day.